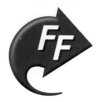

Fast Facts

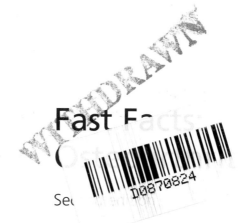

Fast Facts

Osteoarthritis

Second edition

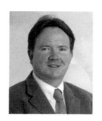

Philip G Conaghan MB BS PhD FRACP FRCP
Professor of Musculoskeletal Medicine
University of Leeds
Consultant Rheumatologist
Leeds Teaching Hospitals NHS Trust &
National Institute for Health Research (NIHR)
Leeds Musculoskeletal Biomedical Research Unit
Leeds, West Yorkshire, UK

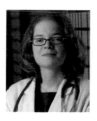

Amanda E Nelson MD MSCR
Assistant Professor of Medicine
Division of Rheumatology, Allergy, and Immunology
University of North Carolina
Thurston Arthritis Research Center
Chapel Hill, North Carolina, USA

Declaration of Independence
This book is as balanced and as practical as we can make it.
Ideas for improvement are always welcome: feedback@fastfacts.com

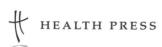

HEALTH PRESS

Fast Facts: Osteoarthritis
First published 2009
Second edition April 2012

Text © 2012 Philip G Conaghan, Amanda E Nelson
© 2012 in this edition Health Press Limited

Health Press Limited, Elizabeth House, Queen Street, Abingdon,
Oxford OX14 3LN, UK
Tel: +44 (0)1235 523233
Fax: +44 (0)1235 523238

Book orders can be placed by telephone or via the website.
For regional distributors or to order via the website, please go to:
www.fastfacts.com
For telephone orders, please call +44 (0)1752 202301 (UK, Europe and Asia–
Pacific), 1 800 247 6553 (USA, toll free) or +1 419 281 1802 (Americas).

Fast Facts is a trademark of Health Press Limited.

A CIP record for this title is available from the British Library.

ISBN 978-1-908541-09-3

Conaghan PG (Philip)
Fast Facts: Osteoarthritis/
Philip G Conaghan, Amanda E Nelson

Medical illustrations by Dee McLean, London, UK.
Typesetting and page layout by Zed, Oxford, UK.
Printed by Latimer Trend & Company Limited, Plymouth, UK.

Text printed with vegetable inks on biodegradable and
recyclable paper manufactured from sustainable forests.

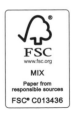

FSC
www.fsc.org
MIX
Paper from
responsible sources
FSC® C013436

Introduction

Osteoarthritis (OA) represents a massive and growing problem for our aging and overweight society: all health professionals reading this book will have encountered OA in the clinic, if not personally. *Fast Facts: Osteoarthritis* provides an up-to-date, clinically relevant, all-in-one reference for all providers caring for individuals with OA.

For most people, OA is a syndrome of joint pain and stiffness with associated functional problems that have a substantial effect on quality of life. In terms of structural abnormalities, OA is best thought of as joint 'failure', just as we consider other age-related organ failures. However, the distinction between symptomatic and structural (often radiographic) evidence of OA is worth considering when evaluating the OA literature, as there is often a discordant relationship between the presence of symptoms and radiographic findings.

The OA process has been recognized since ancient times, affecting both humans and animals, and is strongly associated with age and trauma. Research is constantly under way to better understand the OA process and to develop new therapeutic approaches. The use of MRI and, increasingly, ultrasound in OA research has already begun to affect our understanding of structural features such as synovitis and bone marrow lesions associated with both pain and disease progression.

From the treatment strategies currently available, including patient education and support, pain relief and surgical intervention, it is important that management plans are tailored to individual patients' needs, enabling them to lead active and productive lives. This second edition of *Fast Facts: Osteoarthritis* includes comprehensive updates, including new information on epidemiology, risk factors, and pharmacological as well as non-pharmacological treatments.

Although there is no cure for OA, for those clinicians who find it challenging to deal with people's OA pain, we hope this new edition provides support for our view that **something can be done to help every person with OA**.

The normal joint

An understanding of the key structures in the normal joint
(Figure 1.1), including their composition and function, is a prerequisite
for understanding any arthritic process.

Articular cartilage

The end of each bone within a joint is lined with hyaline cartilage.
Normal articular hyaline cartilage varies in thickness at different sites,
not only within a given joint but at the same site between individuals,
possibly between men and women and at different ages. The only cells
in cartilage are chondrocytes. These cells are rather sparse, making up
less than 5% of the tissue volume, and their density decreases with

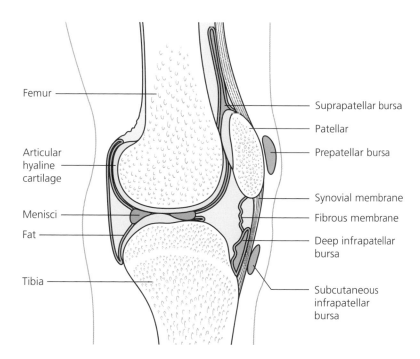

Figure 1.1 Lateral view of a normal knee joint.

distance from the joint cavity. Cartilage tissue is largely composed of an extracellular matrix that is produced by the chondrocytes. This matrix is very well hydrated, consisting of 70–80% water, protein collagen fibers, proteoglycans, glycosaminoglycans and some non-collagen proteins (Figure 1.2). Articular cartilage has no blood vessels, lymphatics or nerves, so the chondrocytes receive nutrition by diffusion of molecules from the synovial fluid in the joint cavity through the extracellular matrix.

Histologically, the cartilage is seen as an upper non-calcified layer divided into the following zones:

- superficial, with few cells and tangential collagen fibers (zone I)
- intermediate, with oblique fiber orientation (zone II)
- deep, with vertical fibers (zone III).

These zones are separated from the deeper calcified cartilage (zone IV) abutting subchondral bone by a basophilic-staining tidemark, the point at which the cartilage starts to become calcified (Figures 1.2 and 1.3).

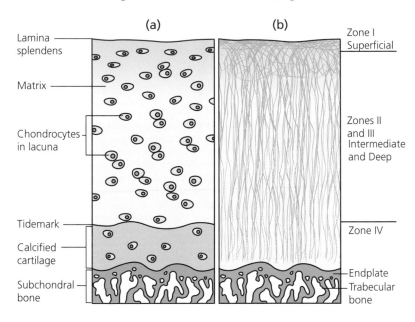

Figure 1.2 Composition and structure of normal articular hyaline cartilage and subchondral bone, showing (a) the histology and (b) the orientation of the collagen fibers.

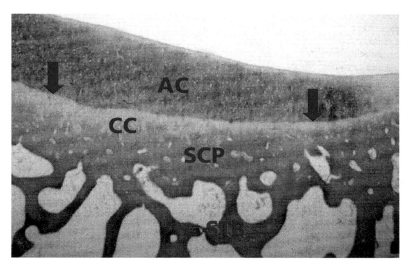

Figure 1.3 Histological section showing the structure of a normal joint. The articular cartilage (AC) is separated from the calcified cartilage (CC) by the tidemark (arrows; see Figure 1.2). The calcified cartilage forms an irregular boundary with the underlying subchondral bone plate (SCP), while the SCP is architecturally distinct from subchondral trabecular bone (STB). Reproduced with permission of Elsevier. All rights reserved. Copyright © 2003 Burr DB. *Osteoarthritis Cartilage* 2004;12:S20–S30.

The collagen fibers of the extracellular matrix give tensile strength and three-dimensional shape to the cartilage. The fibers are composed of compact, triple-helical collagen molecules (Figure 1.4), which are classified according to length and side chains: collagen type II makes up 80–90% of the articular cartilage collagen.

Proteoglycans are complex, specialized macromolecules with a linear protein core and covalently attached glycosaminoglycan side chains. Aggrecan is the major proteoglycan of articular cartilage and has a protein core with glycosaminoglycan side-chains of keratan sulfate and chondroitin sulfate (Figure 1.5). These glycosaminoglycans are linear chains of repeating polysaccharide subunits. The aggrecan molecules in the extracellular matrix are stabilized by link protein and are attached to hyaluronic acid (HA) molecules, which are also very large glycosaminoglycans. One HA molecule may bind up to

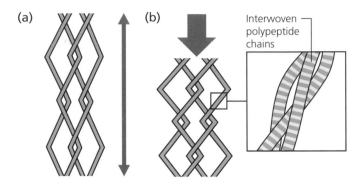

Figure 1.4 The collagen fiber network of articular hyaline cartilage, showing (a) strength under tension, and (b) the ability to withstand compression. Inset: each fiber is composed of three helical collagen molecules (see Figure 1.5).

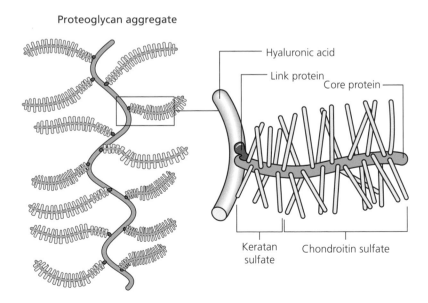

Figure 1.5 The structure of the proteoglycan (PG) molecule and PG aggregate.

200 aggrecan molecules, forming a macromolecular aggregate (see Figure 1.5). Aggrecan gives cartilage its elastic properties in circumstances of compressive load. Tissue loading results in changes in the degree of hydration of aggrecan in the extracellular matrix (via the hydrophilic glycosaminoglycan chains). Proteoglycans have an average half-life of approximately 25 days, compared with at least a few years for type II collagen.

The roles of other, less abundant, non-collagenous proteins in the extracellular matrix, including cartilage oligomeric matrix protein, decorin, lumican and biglycan, are less fully understood.

Normal cartilage homeostasis requires a balance between the synthesis and degradation of components in the extracellular matrix, both by chondrocytes and by the actions of various soluble mediators derived from the chondrocytes and synovium (Table 1.1). The metalloproteinases are the most important in the degradation of type II collagen and aggrecan. These include the matrix metalloproteinases (MMPs) and ADAMTS proteases (disintegrin and metalloproteinases with thrombospondin motifs, some of which are also known as aggrecanases). The activity of these metalloproteinases increases in the presence of the cytokines interleukin (IL)-1 and tumor necrosis factor (TNF)α. Cytokine regulators include the IL-1 receptor antagonist (IL-1RA) and the human cytokine synthesis inhibitory factor IL-10. MMP activity is modulated by naturally occurring inhibitors known as tissue inhibitors of matrix metalloproteinase (TIMPs). Mechanical loading increases proteoglycan production by chondrocytes. This classification of catabolic and anabolic effects of various molecules is somewhat simplistic; it is important to understand that such molecules may have complex augmenting and/or antagonizing effects in vivo, such as those of nitric oxide species and the Wnt pathway.

Subchondral bone

The lower levels of the cartilage away from the joint cavity become calcified at a point called the tidemark (see Figures 1.2 and 1.3); the region extending from this calcified cartilage to the bone marrow is referred to as the subchondral bone and comprises a subchondral plate

TABLE 1.1

The balance between degradation and synthesis in normal cartilage homeostasis

Degradative/catabolic factors

- Cytokines: IL-1, TNFα, LIF
- Proteinases:
  - Cysteine (e.g. cathepsin K) and serine proteinases (e.g. plasmin, plasminogen activators)
  - Metalloproteinases: MMP-1 (interstitial collagenase), MMP-2 (gelatinase), MMP-3 (stromelysin), MMP-13 (collagenase-3); ADAMTS-4 and -5 (aggrecanase-1 and -2)
  - Dickkopf-related protein 1 (DKK-1)

Pro-synthesis/anabolic factors

- Cytokine inhibitors/regulators: IL-1RA, IL-10
- Proteinase inhibitor: TIMP
- Growth factors: FGF, EGF, TGFβ, bone morphogenetic proteins
- Mechanical loading (increases proteoglycan production by chondrocytes)

ADAMTS, a disintegrin and a metalloproteinase with thrombospondin motifs; EGF, epidermal growth factor; FGF, fibroblast growth factor; IL, interleukin; IL-1RA, IL-1 receptor antagonist; LIF, leukemia inhibitory factor; MMP, matrix metalloproteinase; TGFβ, transforming growth factor β; TIMP, tissue inhibitor of MMP; TNFα, tumor necrosis factor α.

and underlying trabecular bone. The subchondral bone is therefore intimately associated with the overlying cartilage and probably acts as a single structure for load transmission. Like cartilage, the thickness of the subchondral bone may vary with age and location within a joint; it may be thicker in the central weight-bearing areas of joints. The calcified cartilage layer is of intermediate stiffness between overlying cartilage and subchondral bone. The subchondral bone has a density similar to cortical bone but the trabeculae are aligned in different directions, resulting in different mechanical properties depending on the plane of loading.

The cellular elements of bone are the osteoblasts, which are of mesenchymal cell origin and produce collagen and bone matrix, and the osteoclasts, which appear to be marrow-derived macrophage-like cells responsible for bone resorption. The bone matrix is composed primarily of inorganic mineral, with about 25% comprising organic matrix and cells. Type I collagen is the major organic component of bone. The type I collagen molecules are cross-linked by molecules such as pyridinoline. Bone mineral is generally referred to as hydroxyapatite. Non-collagenous proteins present in the matrix include proteoglycans, osteocalcin and bone sialoprotein.

The subchondral bone has an abundant vascular supply with extensive vascular anastomoses between the vessels. These vessels are important in maintaining homeostasis of the subchondral bone via remodeling. Nerve fibers have also been demonstrated in the Haversian canals of the subchondral bone.

Normal bone homeostasis. Like cartilage, bone homeostasis is a complex but tightly controlled process involving a balance between pro-synthetic and resorptive factors. Bone remodeling is influenced by various factors, including genetics, hormones (e.g. sex steroids, parathyroid hormone, growth factors), vitamin D, biomechanics (mechanotransducers within bone cells respond to stresses across the bone) and the environment (poor calcium intake, excessive alcohol intake and cigarette smoking are risk factors for reduced bone mass). Later in life the resorptive factors dominate, resulting in a high prevalence (greater than 30%) of osteoporosis in individuals over 65 years of age (see *Fast Facts: Osteoporosis*).

Menisci

The fibrocartilaginous menisci are generally associated with the knee joint, but are also found in other sites such as the sternoclavicular and temporomandibular joints. The menisci of the knee are crescent-shaped tissues that lie between the medial and lateral tibiofemoral joint surfaces. They function to distribute and attenuate load, and contribute to joint stability, proprioception and lubrication. The peripheral portion of the knee meniscus is vascularized and innervated, whereas the inner two-thirds is avascular and aneural, with chondrocytes surrounded by an extracellular matrix comprised of predominantly type I collagen as well as proteoglycans such as chondroitin sulfate. Repair and remodeling appear possible in the peripheral zone of the menisci.

Synovium

The synovium is a membrane that forms the inner lining of the joint cavity but does not cover the articular cartilage. Healthy joints contain a small amount of synovial fluid (see below), a lubricating liquid that supplies nutrients and oxygen to the cartilage. The synovium consists of an intimal or lining layer and a subintimal layer. The intimal layer contains two cell types, or synoviocytes (described below), which form a tight extracellular matrix by interdigitation of cell processes; the subintimal layer comprises connective tissue, which may be areolar, fibrous or adipose. The synovium may form folds and also projections called villi.

In humans, the thickness of the subintimal layer varies in depth, from 100 μm to 5 mm, at given sites within an individual. By contrast, the lining layer is generally one or two cells (25–35 μm) in thickness. Although information is limited, the structure of the synovium does not appear to undergo any major changes with aging.

Synoviocytes within the intimal lining layer are classified ultrastructurally as macrophage-like (type A) or fibroblast-like (type B). Type A cells make up to a third of the intimal cells in normal synovium; these macrophages are derived from the bone marrow and produce the cytokines IL-1 and TNFα, as well as other macrophage-specific products. Type B cells are functionally specialized compared with fibroblasts from other sites. For example, they demonstrate high levels of enzymes required for HA synthesis, and show prominent expression of CD44 (an HA receptor). These synovial fibroblasts are involved in the production of HA, extracellular matrix protein and adhesion molecules, and also in the production of cytokines (including IL-6 and IL-8), arachidonic acid derivatives, growth factors and MMPs. Mechanical factors and surface shearing stress may be important determinants of fibroblast phenotype at connective tissue surfaces.

The synovial intimal extracellular matrix is composed largely of HA, chondroitin sulfates, heparan sulfate, keratan sulfate, collagen (types III–VI), fibronectin and laminin. Interactions between synoviocytes and the extracellular matrix play an important role in the maintenance of the intimal lining layer. Small numbers of antigen-presenting dendritic cells and mast cells are also found in the synovium. The normal synovium is well supplied with blood vessels, which supply nutrition to the intima and nearby cartilage, and nerves, which often extend to the intimal layer.

The synovial fluid lies within the synovial cavity; molecules and cells pass in and out of the synovial fluid passage via the synovial intima and its underlying microcirculation. The intimal matrix has a sieve-like role, allowing diffusion of water and other small molecules while preventing the rapid movement of large molecules such as albumin and HA.

The synovial fluid is largely composed of an ultrafiltrate of plasma (except for the HA concentration). Its major non-cellular constituents are HA and proteins of relatively low molecular weight such as albumin and B globulins. It may also contain small numbers of leukocytes.

Synovial fluid is highly viscous and its volume varies from joint to joint; normal values are not well defined. The synovial intimal cells regulate the volume of synovial fluid, largely by control of HA production. Up to 3 mL of synovial fluid have been aspirated from normal human knee joints, and these volumes may increase during exercise.

Key points – the normal joint

- The complex joint structure provides frictionless articulation and load-bearing abilities.
- The joint should be seen as a single dynamic structure with inter-relating components.

Key references

Compston JE, Rosen CJ. *Fast Facts: Osteoporosis*, 6th edn. Oxford: Health Press Limited, 2009.

Klippel JH, Dieppe PA, eds. *Rheumatology*, 2nd edn. London: Mosby, 1998.

Simkin PA, Gardner GC. The musculoskeletal system and joint physiology. In: Hochberg MC, Silman AJ, Smolen JS et al., eds. *Rheumatology*, 4th edn. Mosby-Elsevier, 2008:33–43.

The dysregulated osteoarthritis (OA) process involves all the tissues within the joint. This chapter focuses on the pathological findings in the cartilage, subchondral bone, menisci and synovium of the OA joint.

Articular cartilage

The early changes in cartilage degradation are those of increased hydration along with progressive breakdown of the collagen fibrillar network, especially due to denaturation of type II collagen. Later, there are areas of both replication and death of chondrocytes, disruption to the cartilage surface with the formation of fibrillated areas and clefts, and evidence of vascular invasion into the calcified cartilage zone (Figure 2.1).

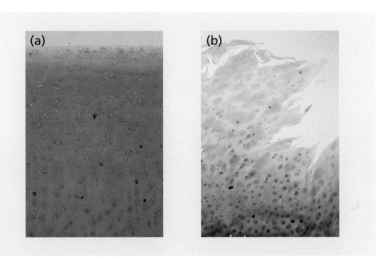

Figure 2.1 Histological sections of cartilage from (a) a normal joint with a smooth surface and (b) an OA joint in which the collagen network has degenerated, resulting in the formation of fibrillated areas and clefts on the surface and loss of staining for proteoglycans. Reproduced with permission of BioMed Central, from Mastbergen et al. *Arthritis Res Ther* 2006;8:R2.

The metabolism of cartilage changes dramatically. Initially, perhaps in an attempt at repair, the chondrocytes become more active and increase the synthesis of proteoglycans, but ultimately there is net loss of proteoglycan from the matrix. There are also changes in proteoglycan structure, in that the aggrecan monomers are smaller and have diminished ability to associate with hyaluronic acid. The loss of proteoglycan parallels the disease severity and these structural changes may account for the failure of matrix repair.

The enzymes produced by cartilage and synovium, described in normal cartilage homeostasis (see Table 1.1, page 12), play a major role in the breakdown of cartilage in OA. The matrix metalloproteinases (MMPs) in particular have been studied extensively. Collagenase (MMP-3) breaks down the triple-helical structure of type II collagen and removes pro-peptide elements important in fibril formation. It can also cleave type X collagen but not the minor collagens. Stromelysin (MMP-13) cleaves aggrecan but can also degrade collagens type VI, IX and XI. Increased levels of MMP have been demonstrated in OA cartilage compared with normal cartilage, particularly in the upper zones. The relative proportions of MMPs and tissue inhibitors of MMP (TIMPs) are also altered in OA cartilage. The relative importance of MMPs and aggrecanases (ADAMTS) is still not fully understood.

Other proteases also play a role in cartilage breakdown, directly or indirectly. After interleukin (IL)-1 stimulation, chondrocytes produce the serine proteases known as plasminogen activators, which subsequently increase the levels of plasmin. Plasmin may act indirectly in cartilage degradation by activating MMPs.

As demonstrated in Figure 2.2, cytokines also play a major role in cartilage homeostasis and are also important in driving the OA process. The synovium seems to be the major source of these cytokines (see pages 20–2). Importantly, OA cartilage seems to be more susceptible to pro-inflammatory cytokines IL-1 and tumor necrosis factor (TNF)α, and upregulation of TNFα receptors has been demonstrated in OA chondrocytes. Differences in the numbers of cytokine receptors have also been demonstrated in chondrocytes from different sites, perhaps accounting for the often focal nature of cartilage defects.

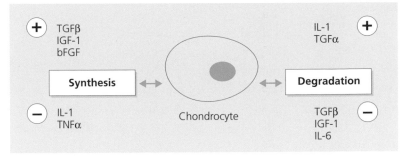

Figure 2.2 Influence of cytokines on cartilage matrix synthesis and degradation. bFGF, basic fibroblast growth factor; IGF, insulin-like growth factor; IL, interleukin; TGF, transforming growth factor; TNF, tumor necrosis factor.

Subchondral bone

The well-described bony features of OA are generally those of exposed, or cartilage-denuded, subchondral bone: macroscopically this has a polished marble appearance (eburnation), while microscopically the bone is thickened (sclerotic) with cystic defects (Figure 2.3). In non-weight-bearing marginal areas, overgrowths of bone, called osteophytes, develop, which may represent an attempt by bone to cope with the abnormal loading and stress associated with pathology such as cartilage loss.

Changes in subchondral bone may arise from changes in bone vascularity. Increased expression of vascular endothelial growth factor (VEGF) may contribute to increased bone and cartilage angiogenesis and vascularity in OA. Changes in blood-flow distribution have been described in subchondral bone, with marrow hypertension and edema. The associated vascular congestion leads to acidosis and hypoxia, which may contribute to the bony pathology. The causes of vascular congestion are not fully understood but pro-thrombotic defects have been detected in studies of patients with primary OA, suggesting a hypercoagulable state with hypofibrinolysis and hyperlipidemia. MRI changes in bone are described later in this chapter.

Menisci

The menisci have only recently become a focus for OA research, and they probably play a crucial role in OA pathogenesis, both as a cause

(a)   (b)

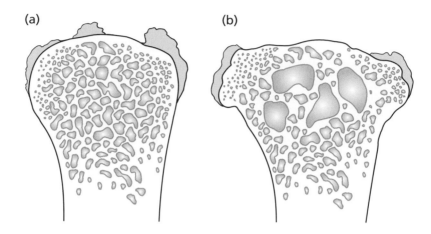

Figure 2.3 As the disease progresses (a) patchy loss of articular cartilage exposes the subchondral bone beneath (eburnation); (b) extensive loss of cartilage results in changes in the bone itself, including fibrosis, cystic degeneration and osteophyte formation.

and as a consequence of the disease process. MRI studies are improving our understanding of the pathogenic role of menisci (see pages 26–8).

Meniscal damage and tears, as well as some degree of meniscal extrusion, are very common in established OA. The relative avascularity of the inner two-thirds of the meniscus means that it is unable to repair, with normalization of structure, after initial injury. Removal of the meniscus post-injury leads to increased risk of OA, and more conservative meniscal repair procedures, although imperfect, are currently advocated. Perimeniscal synovitis is frequent in advanced OA, where complete degeneration or maceration of the meniscus is also common.

Synovium

Synovitis – inflammation of the synovium – occurs with increasing frequency with progressive severity of OA. Studies of biopsies taken at the time of joint-replacement surgery (i.e. at a severe stage of OA) have shown a very high incidence of synovitis. A study using ultrasonography in 600 people with painful knee OA demonstrated synovial inflammation or effusion in almost half the population, despite using a strict definition of synovial hypertrophy.

Researchers have also demonstrated the existence of synovitis even in early clinical disease. In a group of relatively young patients with arthroscopically proven OA but minimal radiological evidence of disease, 29 (mean age 40) were investigated for knee pain and 14 (mean age 24) for joint instability. Approximately half in each group had microscopic evidence of synovitis.

Causes of synovitis. Clues as to the factors that may cause, or at least influence, the presence of synovitis have largely arisen from analysis of synovial fluid. In most cases, the synovial fluid in OA contains an elevated number of leukocytes, although not as markedly increased as in rheumatoid arthritis (RA). Most of these cells are neutrophils, which are not usually found in synovium. IL-8, which is found in OA synovial fluid, is produced by both synovial macrophages and synovial fibroblasts in response to IL-1, and may be the responsible chemoattractant. The cytokines IL-1, IL-6, TNFα, prostaglandin E2 and fibroblast growth factor (FGF) have also been found in the synovial fluid. Elevated nitrite and nitrate levels provide evidence for the production of nitric oxide, an important pro-inflammatory reactive oxygen species.

Synovial fluid in OA also often contains cartilage fragments, calcium pyrophosphate dihydrate (CPPD) and apatite crystals, and elevated levels of cartilage matrix macromolecules. These breakdown products of articular cartilage may be an important cause of synovial inflammation. Cartilage fragments or shards have been reported in OA synovial tissue as well as fluid, but macroscopic fragments are probably not as important as extracellular-matrix macromolecules in promoting synovial inflammation.

Chondroitin sulfate, type II collagen, cartilage proteoglycans and homogenized cartilage have all been shown to produce synovial inflammation in animal models. An autosensitization process is also suggested by the presence of autoantibodies to native and denatured type II collagen found in OA cartilage, immunoglobulin–complement complexes demonstrated in superficial OA cartilage and terminal complement components demonstrated in OA synovium.

CPPD and apatite crystals are also seen in synovial biopsies and radiographs (chondrocalcinosis) and, again, become more prevalent with increasing disease severity. In general, the presence of these crystals has not been correlated with clinical signs of inflammation but they do induce cytokine (especially IL-1) production and consequently inflammation.

Histological changes of synovitis in patients with OA are different from those seen in patients with RA by a matter of degree. In OA synovitis, the thickness of the lining layer increases, angiogenesis increases, and mononuclear and plasma-cell cellular infiltration occurs. Both B and T lymphocytes are present in OA synovium, with the CD4-positive subset predominating (as in RA). Cytotoxic T cells and natural killer cells, both of which contain serine proteinases, have been demonstrated in OA synovium.

Elevated levels of cytokines (e.g. IL-1α, IL-1β, TNFα) and MMPs have been demonstrated in OA tissue; although these cytokines are also produced by chondrocytes, the synovium is thought to be the major site of production. As expected in any biological system, levels of natural cytokine inhibitors (IL-1 receptor antagonist proteins and TIMPs) are elevated in human OA synovium (compared with non-arthritic tissue). Other important inflammatory molecules upregulated in OA synovium include adhesion molecules, granulocyte and granulocyte-macrophage colony-stimulating factors, and the neuropeptide substance P, which is pro-inflammatory and stimulates IL-1 secretion.

Functional joint pathology

It is not sufficient to merely describe the pathological features of individual tissues in the OA joint without considering the pathology of the joint as a functional unit, where a complex interplay of periarticular muscles, joint alignment, ligamentous strength and intra-articular pathology occurs.

Malalignment of the knee increases load through the medial compartment in the varus knee. Associations with both increased medial bone mineral density and bone-marrow edema on MRI have been described. Knee alignment influences structural progression at both the tibiofemoral and patellofemoral joints. Gait analyses suggest that the most important force through the knee is the adduction moment, which produces medial joint force in knees with a varus deformity (Figure 2.4). This adduction moment is negatively correlated with the width of the medial joint space. Differences in gait have been demonstrated between normal subjects and those with mild or severe (radiographic) OA. Patterns of varus and valgus thrust (dynamic malalignment) may specifically predispose to medial and lateral knee OA, respectively.

Periarticular muscles may become weaker as a consequence of OA pain; conversely, weak periarticular muscles may be a risk factor for the development of OA. In medial OA of the knee, there may be greater co-contraction of medial muscle, resulting in higher joint compression forces. Importantly, recent work has highlighted the frequency of knee instability in patients with knee OA, with effects on function beyond that expected from pain, reduced range of movement and quadriceps strength.

Radiographic pathology

Radiography has been the long-established method for evaluating in-vivo pathology in OA. As discussed in Chapter 3, there is often a discordant relationship between the presence of symptoms and radiographic findings. The classic radiographic findings (Figures 2.5–2.7) are:

- joint-space narrowing, which represents a combination of hyaline cartilage loss and meniscal degeneration/extrusion
- osteophytes (bony spurs)
- subchondral bone thickening (sclerosis)
- subchondral bone cyst formation.

Chondrocalcinosis, or calcification of areas of the hyaline cartilage, may also be seen. Calcium crystals are commonly seen in joint aspirates from OA joints, and recent work looking at joint-replacement tissue suggests that calcification is extremely common in joints with end-stage OA.

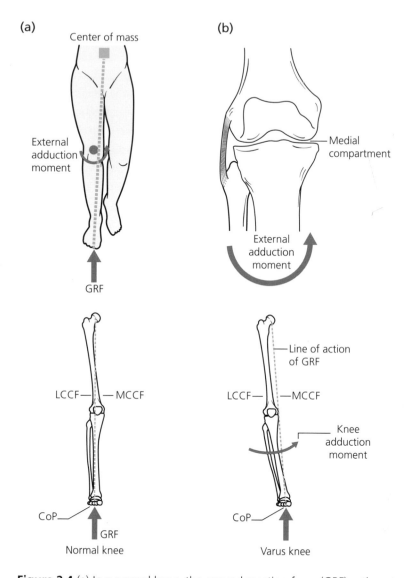

Figure 2.4 (a) In a normal knee, the ground reaction force (GRF) acting at the center of pressure (CoP) of the foot will cause near equal magnitudes of lateral compartment compression force (LCCF) and medial compartment compression force (MCCF) within the knee. (b) In a varus knee, the medial shift of the foot and CoP relative to the femur will cause a large increase in the knee adduction moment and an increase in the MCCF, which will, in turn, tend to cause medial compartment OA.

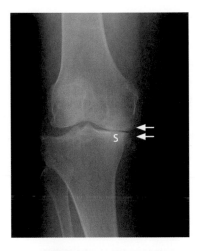

Figure 2.5 Anterior–posterior radiograph of a knee joint with OA. There is marked narrowing of the medial joint space, with osteophyte formation (arrows), and subchondral sclerosis (S).

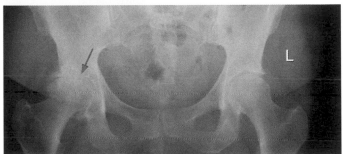

Figure 2.6 Radiograph of a pelvis demonstrating normal left hip (L) and OA of the right hip with loss of joint space (red arrow), especially superiorly, and deformity of the femoral head.

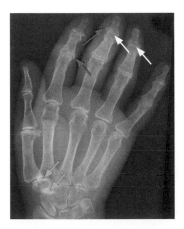

Figure 2.7 Radiograph of a right hand demonstrating OA of the distal and proximal interphalangeal joints, with joint space loss (white arrows) and osteophyte formation (red arrows). There is also OA change (periarticular bony sclerosis) at the first carpometacarpal joint (blue arrows).

25

MRI pathology

Recent MRI studies have helped our understanding of the extent and complexity of OA pathology. MRI enables a three-dimensional evaluation of the joint and allows bone, cartilage and soft tissue to be visualized. However, studies using MRI require careful interpretation because of possible differences in methods used, such as different magnet strengths (e.g. 1.5T vs 0.2T) or different sequences (e.g. if fat suppression is used in order to visualize bone-marrow edema).

Early OA MRI studies focused on assessment of cartilage (since one of the great strengths of MRI above conventional radiographs is the direct detection and quantification of cartilage), but recent studies have included assessment of multiple intra-articular features. These studies have confirmed common abnormalities of most of the tissues in the painful OA joint, demonstrating not only cartilage thinning and loss but also bone-marrow lesions, synovitis, meniscal damage and extrusion, and ligament abnormalities (Figures 2.8–2.10).

Using MRI, approximately half of elderly people with normal knee radiographs are found to have joint abnormalities. Of course, many abnormalities will not be associated with symptoms. The prevalence of most MRI abnormalities increases with age, and cartilage defects are usually modestly correlated with the presence of other (e.g. subchondral bone) abnormalities. In general, abnormalities of multiple structures are more common in painful OA knees than non-painful knees, although this may not be true for the patellofemoral joint.

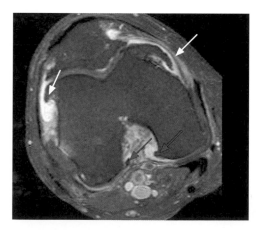

Figure 2.8 Axial MRI scan showing OA of the knee, with large osteophytes on the femoral sides of the patellofemoral joint (white arrows) and small posterior osteophytes in the intercondylar region (red arrows).

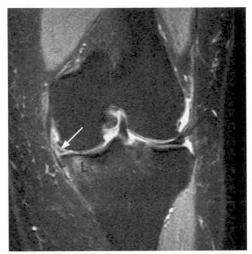

Figure 2.9 Coronal MRI scan of an OA knee, with fat-suppressed sequence highlighting a large bone-marrow lesion in the medial tibial plateau (L). The adjacent medial meniscus is degenerate (white arrow) and can be compared with the more normal appearance of the lateral meniscus (red arrow).

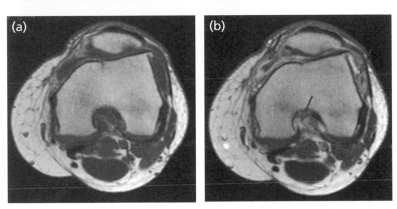

Figure 2.10 T1-weighted axial MRI scans of an OA knee (a) before and (b) after injection of the contrast agent gadolinium, enhancing areas of synovitis (red arrows). MRI scans courtesy of Dr Andrew Grainger, Leeds, UK.

MRI has also provided novel insights into the role of bone in OA. Although there are few histological correlation studies, some of the bone-marrow lesions visualized on MRI represent histological bone-marrow necrosis, fibrosis and abnormally remodeled trabeculae. With respect to structural progression of OA, normal (or negative) bone scintigraphy predicts little, if any, change in joint-space width in the OA knee at follow-up. As a correlate to this, strong associations between bone-marrow lesions and subsequent progression of joint-space narrowing and cartilage loss in the same joint compartment have been reported. The correlation between pain and MRI features is discussed on page 46.

Key points – the OA joint

- All tissues of the joint may show pathology, including cartilage, subchondral bone, the menisci and the synovium.
- The joint should be considered a functional organ, with gait, periarticular muscles and related mechanical forces all playing a role in pathology.
- Modern imaging has highlighted the extensive nature of the pathology, even in joints with limited radiographic evidence of damage.

Key references

Brandt KD, Radin EL, Dieppe PA, van de Putte L. Yet more evidence that osteoarthritis is not a cartilage disease. *Ann Rheum Dis* 2006;65: 1261–4.

Burr D. The importance of the subchondral bone in the progression of osteoarthritis. *J Rheumatol* 2004 (suppl);70:77–80.

Conaghan PG. Is MRI useful in osteoarthritis? *Best Pract Clin Rheumatol* 2006;20:57–68.

D'Agostino MA, Conaghan PG, Le Bars M et al. EULAR report on the use of ultrasonography in painful knee osteoarthritis. Part 1: prevalence of inflammation in osteoarthritis. *Ann Rheum Dis* 2005;64:1703–9.

Englund M, Guermazi A, Lohmander LS. The meniscus in knee osteoarthritis. *Rheum Dis Clin North Am* 2009;35:579–90.

Goldring MB, Goldring SR. Osteoarthritis. *J Cell Physiol* 2007;213:626–34.

Mundermann A, Dyrby CO, Andriacchi TP. Secondary gait changes in patients with medial compartment knee osteoarthritis. *Arthritis Rheum* 2005;52:2835–44.

Myers SL, Brandt KD, Ehlich JW et al. Synovial inflammation in patients with early osteoarthritis of the knee. *J Rheumatol* 1990;17: 1662–9.

Osteoarthritis (OA) is the most common joint disorder and represents a major cause of pain and disability for the individual, as well as resulting in enormous health expenditure in Western countries. In the UK and USA, an estimated 8.5 million and 27 million people are affected by the disorder, respectively. The joints most commonly affected are the:

- hands: base of thumb, distal and proximal interphalangeal joints
- spine: cervical and lumbosacral
- hips
- knees
- first metatarsophalangeal joint.

Definition

OA is not an acquired disease in the traditional medical model, and definitions have not always been clear. As stated in the Introduction, OA is a syndrome of joint pain and stiffness with associated functional problems, which can have a substantial effect on quality of life. In terms of structural abnormalities, OA encompasses a number of problems that result in common pathological and radiological features. The OA disease process in synovial joints is classically characterized in its later stages by focal cartilage degradation, involvement of the subchondral bone and synovium, and the formation of marginal osteophytes; in reality, all components of the joint are affected. Importantly, periarticular tissue, especially muscle, is often affected as well.

Prevalence

Estimates of incidence and prevalence vary according to the definition of OA used; for example, symptomatic versus radiographic criteria. Even when radiographic definitions are used, different radiographic features may be emphasized (e.g. osteophytes vs joint-space narrowing). It is interesting to note that the correlation between pain and radiographic OA features is not as strong as expected, for reasons discussed in Chapter 4 (see pages 45–6).

Radiographic OA is more common than symptomatic OA, and detection rates in a given joint may increase when more radiographic views are obtained. Recent studies on the distribution of radiographic OA have suggested that right-sided hand and knee OA is more common than left-sided disease (consistent with a biomechanical cause). Even within a specific joint, the distribution of osteophytes or joint-space narrowing differs in prevalence, as well as by sex and ethnicity, again reflecting biomechanical and genetic factors (Table 3.1). In the hand, the most common combinations of joints affected by radiographic OA are the distal and proximal interphalangeal joints with or without the carpometacarpal joint. However, because ultrasound can visualize the joint in three dimensions, studies using ultrasound have suggested metacarpophalangeal (MCP) joint OA to be more common than radiographic studies suggest. Knee OA with or without lumbosacral spinal involvement is the most common pattern of large joint involvement.

Effect of age. Individual joints demonstrate a striking age-related rise in the prevalence of radiographic OA. About one-third of all adults have radiographic OA of the hands, with two-thirds over 75 years of age exhibiting OA of the distal interphalangeal joints.

TABLE 3.1

Distribution of osteophytosis prevalence by right knee joint compartment in US adults over 60 years of age

Right knee compartment	Radiographic osteophytosis (%)
Medial tibial	24.2
Lateral tibial	16.6
Medial femoral	13.1
Lateral femoral	11.9

Data from Dillon et al. 2006.

TABLE 3.2

Expected prevalence of knee pain and disability in a practice population of adults aged 55+

	Number with patient characteristic	Number with radiographic evidence of OA
Knee pain and severe disability	160	120*
Knee pain and some disability	1250	730
4 weeks of knee pain in past year	2500	1250
Aged 55+ years	10 000	2510

*Proportion not known but likely to be high. Data estimated from Peat et al., 2001.

Radiographic OA of the knees has also been found in about a third of adults over 60 years of age (Table 3.2).

Effect of sex. The prevalence of radiographic OA (particularly of the hand and knee) is higher in women than men, especially in individuals over 50 years of age.

Effect of ethnicity. The prevalence of large joint radiographic OA in joints other than the hand is higher in African-Americans than in American whites. Ethnic differences have also been demonstrated in (mainland) Chinese people, with the prevalence of hip and hand OA being substantially lower in men and women from Beijing than in US cohorts assessed using the same methods.

Symptomatic OA. Joint pain is common, but not all joint pain is attributable to OA (depending on the definition of OA and extra-articular causes of pain such as tendonitis); indeed, about half of those with radiographic OA report no symptoms. Women report more pain than men, and there are clearly differences in symptoms according to anatomic site (Table 3.3). African-Americans tend to report greater pain and disability compared with Caucasians. Many people have multiple joint pains: a study in individuals over the age of 55 suggested a median number of four painful joints. The most common

31

TABLE 3.3

Percentage estimates of joint pain, swelling and/or stiffness over the past 3 months, lasting for more than 6 weeks, in the population over 55 years of age

Joint pain	Male	Female	Total
Knee	18	25	22
Hands	13	23	19
Feet	14	22	18
Back	13	18	16
Shoulder	13	18	16
Neck	13	17	15
Hip	9	15	13
Elbow	6	7	7

Estimates have been adjusted for age and sex.

combinations of joint pain are knee and foot pain, knee and back pain, and knee and hand pain.

So while knee pain affects about a quarter of the adult population, the prevalence of a painful disabling knee attributable to OA in the UK population over 55 years of age has been estimated at approximately 10%. Current statistics from the USA put the prevalence of a painful OA knee in adults over 45 years of age at 16%. Symptomatic hand OA has a reported prevalence of about 7% in a population-based study, in contrast to the high radiographic incidence, while recent work has suggested that 9.5% of adults in the USA have symptomatic hip OA.

Impact on the individual

OA affects individuals in many complex ways, including:

- symptoms
- loss of function
- restricted participation in activities
- impaired quality of life.

Symptoms. Pain is the commonest reason for patients to present to their family physician; over half of all people with OA say that pain is their worst problem. Patients vary in their descriptions of pain (e.g. sharp, burning, dull ache) and the relationship between pain and activity (e.g. worse on bending knee, worse after prolonged immobility, worse in bed at night). Stiffness is the other major complaint, particularly in relation to hip OA. Often the concepts of pain and stiffness are not clearly distinguished by people with OA.

Loss of function. A detailed survey (the UK OA Nation Report 2004) of over 1700 individuals with OA, with an average of 12 years of symptoms, reported that 81% had constant pain or were limited in performing common daily tasks. Furthermore, when OA pain was 'bad', over half struggled to get out of bed. This last finding is supported by other work that suggests half of people with OA of the knee have significant difficulty with physical function.

These problems are much worse when people have multiple joint pain – for example, people with knee pain alone have three times more difficulty in walking than people without knee pain, but the combination of knee, back and foot pain results in 30 times the difficulty.

Restricted participation in activities. Individuals with OA may report some difficulty with occupational as well as certain leisure activities, depending upon the site and severity of their arthritis. A 2002 survey in the USA found that 1 in 3 adults reported activity limitations because of their arthritis or joint symptoms, with substantial increases predicted over the coming years due to aging and increasing obesity.

Impaired quality of life. People with OA report poor self-esteem, loss of independence and a considerable effect on close relationships. They also report feeling old before their time and perceive themselves to be less healthy than others of the same age (especially if young at the time of diagnosis). Depression, which varies in severity, is common but is not often assessed.

Comorbidities

Studies have suggested that even after adjustment for age, sex and social class, people with OA are at least twice as likely to have comorbid conditions as the general population. Over half the population in some studies demonstrated at least one comorbid condition, including obesity, hypertension or ischemic heart disease. Studies also suggest that the presence of such comorbidities magnifies the impact of OA on the individual. Comorbid conditions may also reduce the effectiveness of therapies.

Although it is difficult to be certain from studies of elderly populations with substantial comorbid medical problems and the potentially adverse effects of polypharmacy, multiple-joint OA may be associated with increased mortality.

Economic impact

Analysis of health statistics and expenditure is extremely difficult, and it is not always possible to discern the costs caused by OA from the costs more often expressed for musculoskeletal diseases as a whole. There are direct costs to health services and indirect costs due to lost productivity; the costs of impaired quality of life are currently impossible to estimate. There is always a time lag of some years in producing these figures because of the size of the OA problem and the resources required to estimate the economic impact of the disease.

Direct costs. In the UK, 2 million adults per year visit their family physician with OA problems, resulting in 3 million consultations per year. The rates of attendance at practitioners' clinics appear to be increasing, even allowing for the aging population, perhaps because of increased public awareness of OA therapies. Over the course of a year there will be approximately 115 000 hospital admissions due to OA. In 2000, over 44 000 hip replacements and over 35 000 knee replacements were performed at a cost of £405 million. Between 1991 and 2006 the number of primary total hip replacements doubled and the number of primary total knee replacements trebled, suggesting a substantial increase in costs, although these figures are not yet available.

> **Key points – epidemiology**
>
> - For most people and clinicians, osteoarthritis (OA) refers to a clinical syndrome of joint pain, functional impairment and impaired quality of life.
> - Although radiographic OA is common, it is not always symptomatic.
> - Joint pain is common, increasingly so with age; individuals frequently have multiple joint pains.
> - OA has a large impact on the individual and society.

The average annual total direct cost to a person with OA (defined by ICD-9 code 715) in the USA in 2000–2004 was estimated at over $10 000, with a total aggregate cost of $23 billion. It is estimated that approximately 570 000 hip replacements and 3.5 million knee replacements will be performed in the USA by 2030, up from 231 000 hip and 542 000 knee replacements in 2006, with the vast majority being done for OA. The total estimated cost of total knee replacements increased by 166% from $5.4 to $14.3 billion between 1998 and 2004, and continues to rise.

Indirect costs. Arthritis-related conditions are the second most common cause of lost working days in the UK. In 1999/2000, 36 million working days were lost through OA alone, at an estimated cost of £3.2 billion in lost productivity. In the same time period, £43 million was spent on community services and £215 million was spent on social services for OA-related problems.

In the USA in 2000, indirect costs were estimated at over $33 billion, while total OA-related costs were in the region of a staggering $60 billion.

And it's getting worse ...

The strong relationship between OA and age means a frightening rapid rise in OA is likely as the 'baby-boomer' generations grow older. The populations of North Americans and Europeans older than

60 have been projected to increase by over 10% by 2050, with this age group making up roughly one-third of the population. As life expectancy increases, it is not surprising that the predicted rates of OA are even more marked for those over 80 years of age. In addition, many Western societies have a substantial and increasing prevalence of obesity, which also increases the OA burden.

Key references

Arthritis Care. OA *Nation Report* 2004. www.arthritiscare.org.uk/ PublicationsandResources/ Forhealthprofessionals/OANation

Arthritis Research Campaign. *Arthritis: The Big Picture*. www. ipsos-mori.com/_assets/polls/2002/ pdf/arthritis.pdf

Culliford DJ, Maskell J, Murray DW et al. Temporal trends in hip and knee replacement in the United Kingdom: 1991 to 2006. *J Bone Joint Surg Br* 2010;92:130–5.

Dillon CF, Rasch EK, Gu Q, Hirsch R. Prevalence of knee osteoarthritis in the United States: arthritis data from the Third National Health and Nutrition Examination Survey 1991–94. *J Rheumatol* 2006;33:2271–9.

Hannan MT, Felson DT, Pincus T. Analysis of the discordance between radiographic changes and knee pain in osteoarthritis of the knee. *J Rheumatol* 2000;27:1513–17.

Keenan AM, Tennant A, Fear J et al. Impact of multiple joint problems on daily living tasks in people in the community over age fifty-five. *Arthritis Rheum* 2006;55:757–64.

Lawrence RC, Felson DT, Helmick CG et al. Estimates of the prevalence of arthritis and other rheumatic conditions in the United States: Part II. *Arthritis Rheum* 2008;58:26–35.

Peat G, McCarney R, Croft P. Knee pain and osteoarthritis in older adults: a review of community burden and current use of primary health care. *Ann Rheum Dis* 2001;60:91–7.

Ricci JA, Stewart WF, Chee E et al. Pain exacerbation as a major source of lost productive time in US workers with arthritis. *Arthritis Rheum* 2005;53:673–81.

United States Bone and Joint Decade. The burden of musculoskeletal diseases in the United States. Rosemont, IL: American Academy of Orthopaedic Surgeons, 2008. Available from www.boneandjointburden.org, last accessed 16 November 2011.

4 Etiology

It is likely that the clinical osteoarthritis (OA) in a given joint represents a common endpoint of multiple insults that result in failure of the joint. Trying to define what causes OA is complicated by factors already alluded to, including the lack of a uniform definition for OA and, in particular, the difficulty of detecting early asymptomatic OA.

As discussed in Chapter 3, joints most commonly affected in humans are the hips, knees, cervical and lumbar spine, the small joints of the hands, base of thumb and base of the great toe. This pattern, together with other observations in humans and animals, has led to one concept of OA as an evolution-related problem, associated with changes in use of joints and grip, walking upright and our relative longevity.

Risk factors

Risk factors for OA can be summarized as those resulting in a generalized predisposition for the disease together with localized biomechanical factors; the importance of each risk factor (and the interplay between factors) differs depending on the anatomic site of OA. Although there is some overlap between risk factor profiles for OA incidence and OA progression, these profiles are not identical.

The factors that have been studied as indicators for radiographic progression of tibiofemoral knee OA are listed in Table 4.1. The first part of this table indicates the 'historical' risk factors, from the era when conventional radiographs, with the knee fully extended, were still being used.

In recent studies, using superior radiographic protocols, two quite potent risk factors for progression have been identified – limb malalignment and the MRI feature of bone-marrow lesions. Increasingly, studies employing MRI are using true cartilage assessments (rather than radiographic surrogates such as joint-space narrowing) and are finding similar predictors of progression or progressive cartilage loss.

TABLE 4.1

Factors associated with radiographic progression of tibiofemoral knee OA

Historical

- Heberden's nodes
- Generalized OA
- Anterior cruciate ligament tears
- Knee pain
- Use of NSAIDs
- Joint effusion
- Knee warmth
- Joint fluid CPPD crystals
- Baseline disease severity
- High serum HA
- Contralateral knee OA
- Low vitamin D intake and serum vitamin D level

- High serum IGF-1
- Increasing serum COMP
- Low levels of inorganic pyrophosphate in joint fluid
- High serum CRP
- Older age
- High knee adduction moment
- Female sex
- Increased body mass index
- Increased bodyweight
- Weight:height ratio
- Self-report of 'bow legs' or 'knock knees' in childhood
- Decreased lower extremity tissue mass

In modern studies

- Limb malalignment (i.e. the hip-knee-ankle angle)
- MRI bone-marrow edema lesions (compartment specific)
- Varus thrust (dynamic malalignment)

- Adduction moment at the knee during gait
- Meniscal damage or total meniscectomy
- Reduced internal hip abduction moment*

*Greater hip abductor strength may protect against knee OA progression. COMP, cartilage oligomeric matrix protein; CPPD, calcium pyrophosphate dihydrate; CRP, C-reactive protein; HA, hyaluronic acid; IGF-1, insulin-like growth factor 1; NSAID, non-steroidal anti-inflammatory drug.

Generalized or systemic susceptibility factors include:

- genetic factors
- obesity
- bone mineral density (BMD)
- female sex/hormones
- nutrition.

Localized or biomechanical factors include:

- physical activity
- joint alignment
- trauma
- elite athletic activity.

Genetic factors. It has been known for a long time that primary OA has a genetic element. For a patient with Heberden's nodes, the mother is twice as likely, and the sister is three times as likely, to demonstrate the same OA changes. A study of female twins suggests a genetic influence of up to 65%, but the complex interaction of genetic and environmental factors is far from understood and despite improved methods, much of this heritability remains unexplained.

Types of rare familial OA have been associated with different mutations in the type II pro-collagen gene (type II collagen is the major structural component of articular cartilage), but these mutations have not been found, and there have been no confirmed loci in most cases of primary generalized OA.

The complexity of the OA phenotype (e.g. by anatomic site, limb alignment, symptomatic, radiographic or MRI features) renders genetic association studies difficult. Well-designed studies with appropriate sample size and replication, in the era of genome wide association studies, have revealed only few consistent findings. A single nucleotide polymorphism in the promoter region of *GDF5* (a gene involved in joint formation) has shown a significant association with knee OA in Asian and white populations. A locus at chromosome 7q22, near several potential candidate genes, was associated with knee and/or hand OA in a European population. These variants have modest effect sizes, and may have most of their impact when they occur in combination.

Obesity. A number of studies have demonstrated an association between increased bodyweight and OA of the knee (clinical and structural), but the association with hip OA is weaker; surprisingly, an association with hand OA may also exist, albeit less robust, suggesting systemic factors other than mechanical loading may be important. The majority of longitudinal studies of obesity in OA relate to incident (new development of) OA, and the cross-sectional studies to OA presence versus absence. Although fewer studies have focused on progression of OA, the association with body mass index appears less clear cut, and may be mediated by malalignment.

Bone mineral density. Older studies have suggested a negative association of osteoporosis with OA, especially at the hip, although many of these studies have been cross-sectional. Studies have suggested a generalized increase in bone mass in women with OA of the hands, adding to theories on the role of subchondral bone in the pathogenesis of OA. However, increased BMD is not translated into a reduced fracture risk, perhaps due to OA-associated locomotor problems. The relationship between BMD and OA progression at the knee has not been fully elucidated. Earlier findings that lower BMD was associated with a greater risk of progression may have been due to confounding by lower levels of physical activity.

Female sex/hormones. As mentioned above, the prevalence of OA increases in women after the menopause. This has led to many studies (most cross-sectional) examining the relationship between hormonal status and OA, with conflicting results. Whether estrogen replacement therapy is protective has also not been fully elucidated.

Nutrition. The mechanisms by which nutrients may affect the development of OA are multiple and may include protection from oxidants such as reactive oxygen species and complex modulation of inflammatory responses. Lower levels of vitamin D (an essential component of normal bone biology) have been associated with a greater risk of knee OA progression in some studies, but the association remains controversial. Some preliminary studies have suggested a relationship between serum lipids and MRI bone-marrow lesions, though the mechanism of the relationship is not clear.

Physical activity. There is good epidemiological evidence, including some longitudinal studies, of association between certain occupations and OA incidence, especially of the hip and knee. For example, those involved in occupations involving knee bending, such as farmers and construction workers, have an increased risk of knee OA. The effect of occupations on OA progression is unknown.

Joint alignment. Static varus alignment of the knee (bow-legged appearance) has been associated with a marked increase in the risk of medial progression of medial compartment knee OA, and valgus alignment (knock-kneed appearance) with lateral progression (Figure 4.1). Dynamic malalignment, as in varus or valgus thrust with walking, may also play a role. Knee joint laxity, especially varus–valgus laxity, may also be associated with accelerated progression. Alterations in bone shape, such as congenital dislocation of the hip, femoroacetabular impingement and epiphyseal dysplasia may also predispose to OA.

Trauma. The knee joint has probably been best studied in this category, especially in athletes in whom repetitive high-weight loading

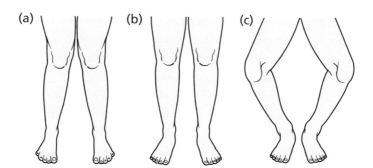

Figure 4.1 (a) Valgus deformity of the knee (also known as 'knock knees'), (b) normal alignment, and (c) varus deformity of the knee (also known as 'bow legs').

is associated with increased rates of OA. A history of joint injury is a significant risk factor for the later development of OA of the knee and also of the hip. At the intra-articular level, both meniscectomy and anterior cruciate ligament tears increase the risk of OA.

Elite athletic activity. Although there are few good longitudinal studies in this area, it appears that athletic activity at the elite level (i.e. national/international competition) is associated with an increased risk of OA after adjusting for injury. Several studies suggest that recreational physical and athletic activity (not at the elite level) does not increase the risk of developing knee OA in a healthy joint.

Etiopathogenesis

Although the pathogenesis of OA remains unknown, current concepts may help explain much of the known OA data and risk factors presented above. Paul Dieppe has proposed a model of OA that encompasses these concepts (Figure 4.2). The normal joint needs both mechanical forces and biochemical remodeling of the cartilage matrix to maintain integrity.

OA is conceptualized as a failed or decompensated remodeling of the joint after an initial injury. The initiating injury may be traumatic (acute or accumulated with time) or occur in tissues made susceptible by the generalized or local factors listed above. Typical injuries may cause meniscal tears, subsequent adjacent cartilage loss, direct chondral or osteochondral defects or ligamentous defects that subsequently lead to meniscal extrusion or abnormal load bearing through the joint. However, it has been demonstrated that not all cartilage lesions result in OA and therefore a second step may occur. This OA process occurs as a result of failed repair or because of abnormal mechanical stimuli or aberrant/overwhelmed biochemical processes. As part of this process, osteophytes will be formed. The clinical expression is further modified, for example, by patient age and sex.

One of the main difficulties in determining the initial or initiating events in OA stems from the fact that individuals do not present with OA until clinical disease is evident and often established or even

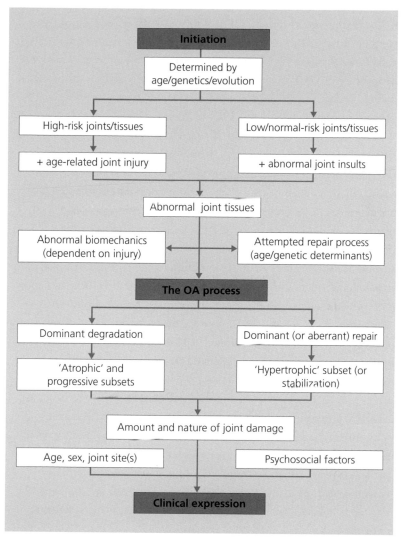

Figure 4.2 Etiopathogenesis of osteoarthritis. Adapted from Dieppe 1995.

advanced. Abnormalities in a number of tissues beyond the cartilage could be involved in OA pathogenesis, and of course these may coexist in an individual.

Researchers have turned to animal models of OA to look for clues to the initiating events, but there is no consensus, and results from animal models must be interpreted with care. Evidence from models in the macaque monkey, the rabbit impulsive loading model and the canine cruciate deficiency model support a pathogenic role for subchondral stiffening. There has been increasing interest in studying post-injury OA, which may provide a window to early, asymptomatic disease and identify potential early diagnostic biomarkers or preventive treatments.

The role of subchondral bone may be important in the initiation of OA. The etiologic concept is that changes in the subchondral bone or cartilage/bone interface lead to an inability of bone to withstand normal mechanical stresses, consequently increasing the stress on overlying cartilage. Clinical studies in women with OA of the hands have looked at bone taken from non-weight-bearing sites distant from the involved joints and have demonstrated a generalized increase in bone mass. Other studies have confirmed increased BMD in patients with generalized OA, and demonstrated quantitative and qualitative changes in the degree of mineralization and growth factor content of bone. Subchondral bone texture, a feature on radiographs measured by a technique called fractal signature analysis, has been shown to predict knee OA progression.

Meniscal damage. In terms of pathogenesis, meniscal damage will cause abnormal loading through the adjacent cartilage (or osteochondral segment) and this has been demonstrated as early cartilage abnormalities on MRI. Meniscal extrusion (related to damage or ligamentous laxity) will also cause abnormal joint loading. In general, medial meniscus damage correlates with varus deformity in the knee.

Ligament abnormalities are commonly associated with OA in MRI studies, and some work in early OA suggests that ligament abnormalities are associated with development of the disease. In addition, primary problems with the periarticular muscles or neuromuscular pathways that provide joint stability have all been linked to OA development, although long-term follow-up studies are lacking.

What causes OA joint pain?

Importantly, the cause of joint pain in OA is not well understood. Pain is a complex and personal phenomenon, and generally a biopsychosocial approach is required to understand an individual's symptoms. This section deals simply with novel concepts of structure–pain relationships as an examination of potential sources of peripheral nociception. It does not attempt to explore other facets of pain, such as spinal or central processing pathways, all of which are important (see *Fast Facts: Chronic and Cancer Pain*).

Possible peripheral sites of pain origin include the:

- synovium
- subchondral bone
- osteophytes
- menisci
- collateral ligaments.

The cartilage is aneural and is therefore unlikely to be the primary source of joint pain (although the cartilage is a source of pro-inflammatory antigens and molecules). Although MRI is superior to radiographs for visualizing osteophytes, MRI studies have not consistently confirmed the relationship between osteophytes and pain suggested by radiographic studies.

Structure–pain studies. Traditional research into structure–pain associations relied on the conventional radiograph, which predominantly images only bone and a surrogate measure of cartilage (the joint space). The vast majority of these radiographic studies have focused on the knee. Such studies are often difficult to interpret because of differences in how the pain was measured (e.g. global pain vs night pain vs weight-bearing pain) and the limitations of conventional radiographs. In addition, many radiographic studies did not include the patellofemoral joint.

One study demonstrated that intra-articular injection of local anesthetic abolished OA knee pain in the majority of (but not all) subjects, suggesting that structures in contact with the intra-articular environment are important in pain production. Stronger associations between radiographic features of knee OA and knee pain have been found using a novel within-person method to reduce confounding, but in general the relationship between radiographic abnormalities and pain is not strong; it is probably stronger when there is more severe radiographic damage. Newer instruments have been designed to assess different facets of the pain experience in OA, such as intermittent versus constant pain (e.g. the measure of Intermittent and Constant Osteoarthritis Pain [ICOAP]).

MRI features associated with OA knee pain. As mentioned in Chapter 2, MRI has improved our understanding of in-vivo pathology in OA. MRI studies have shown the following abnormalities to be associated with knee pain:

- synovitis (i.e. synovial hypertrophy) and effusions
- bone-marrow lesions
- periarticular lesions.

Synovitis and effusions. An association of effusion with pain in OA of the knee has also been suggested in ultrasonography studies, whereas arthroscopy studies (which differ in their ability to visualize and quantify synovitis) have not shown this association. Clearly, this is an important issue for further research as therapies that reduce synovitis may improve pain control.

Bone-marrow lesions. The subchondral bone has been thought to be a source of pain in OA for many years. The presence of large lesions of bone-marrow edema has been associated with pain, and changes in bone-marrow lesions correlate with fluctuations in pain in individuals without evidence of radiographic OA.

Periarticular lesions. Periarticular pathology, including anserine bursitis and iliotibial band syndrome, has been associated with knee pain, perhaps explaining the pain in a small percentage of patients with normal radiographs. There is an important message here for careful clinical examination.

Key points – etiology

- The osteoarthritis (OA) phenotype represents a common endpoint of multiple insults that result in failure of the joint.
- The risk factors differ for incidence and progression.
- There are multiple potential peripheral sources of pain in the pathological OA joint, but the role of spinal and central pain pathways has not been well explored.

Key references

Brandt KD, Dieppe P, Radin EL. Etiopathogenesis of osteoarthritis. *Rheum Dis Clin North Am* 2008;34:531–59.

Conaghan PG. Is MRI useful in osteoarthritis? *Best Pract Clin Rheumatol* 2006;20:57–68.

Cousins MJ, Gallagher RM. *Fast Facts: Chronic and Cancer Pain*, 2nd edn. Oxford: Health Press Limited, 2011.

Dieppe PA. Osteoarthritis and molecular markers. A rheumatologist's perspective. *Acta Orthop Scand Suppl* 1993;266:1–5.

Dieppe PA. Pathogenesis and management of pain in osteoarthritis. *Lancet* 2005;365:965–73.

Felson DT, Lawrence RC, Dieppe PA et al. Osteoarthritis: new insights. Part 1: the disease and its risk factors. *Ann Intern Med* 2000; 133:635–46.

Hunter DJ, Zhang W, Conaghan PG et al. Systematic review of the concurrent and predictive validity of MRI biomarkers in OA. *Osteoarthritis Cartilage* 2011;19:557–88.

Ikegawa S. New gene associations in osteoarthritis: what do they provide, and where are we going? *Curr Opin Rheumatol* 2007;19:429–34.

Issa SN, Sharma L. Epidemiology of osteoarthritis: an update. *Curr Rheumatol Rep* 2006;8:7–15.

Valdes AM, Spector TD. Genetic Epidemiology of hip and knee osteoarthritis. *Nat Rev Rheumatol* 2011;7:23–32.

Osteoarthritis (OA) is usually diagnosed clinically but may require investigations to aid in differential diagnosis or in assessing the degree of structural severity. Like most rheumatologic conditions, composite diagnostic criteria have been established by experts. Formal consensus-agreed criteria for OA of different joints have been developed by the American College of Rheumatology (Figures 5.1–5.3). Such criteria involve clinical, laboratory and radiographic elements, but most population-based studies have not employed such strict criteria. It is important to note that these criteria are good for diagnosis of moderate-to-severe disease but have not been used to identify early OA, something that may well be more important to clinicians.

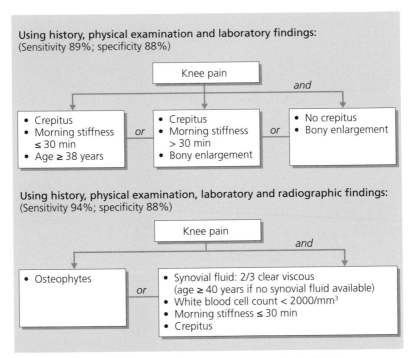

Using history, physical examination and laboratory findings: (Sensitivity 89%; specificity 88%)

Knee pain

and

- Crepitus
- Morning stiffness ≤ 30 min
- Age ≥ 38 years

or

- Crepitus
- Morning stiffness > 30 min
- Bony enlargement

or

- No crepitus
- Bony enlargement

Using history, physical examination, laboratory and radiographic findings: (Sensitivity 94%; specificity 88%)

Knee pain

and

- Osteophytes

or

- Synovial fluid: 2/3 clear viscous (age ≥ 40 years if no synovial fluid available)
- White blood cell count < 2000/mm³
- Morning stiffness ≤ 30 min
- Crepitus

Figure 5.1 Clinical classification criteria for osteoarthritis of the knee, developed by the American College of Rheumatology.

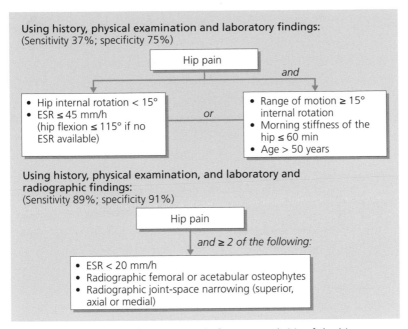

Figure 5.2 Clinical classification criteria for osteoarthritis of the hip, developed by the American College of Rheumatology. ESR, erythrocyte sedimentation rate.

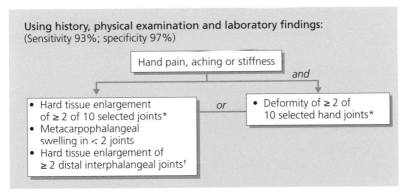

Figure 5.3 Clinical classification criteria for osteoarthritis of the hand, developed by the American College of Rheumatology. *Second and third distal interphalangeal, second and third proximal interphalangeal and first carpometacarpal joints. †The second and third distal interphalangeal joints may be counted both under this category and as one of the ten selected joints described above.

History

When investigating a new patient presenting with any joint problems, it is usual to try to differentiate OA from primary inflammatory arthritides such as rheumatoid arthritis (RA).

Table 5.1 compares the characteristic presenting features of OA with those suggestive of inflammatory arthritis; these form the basis of useful questions to aid diagnosis. The occupational and social history is often useful in determining the 'lifetime load' to which a patient's joints have been exposed. Issues related to diagnoses of the specific joint region are discussed later in this chapter.

Response to anti-inflammatory drugs or intra-articular corticosteroids does not usually help differentiate OA from inflammatory arthritis.

Assessment of joint pain and its consequences. Pain is a complex and personal experience, but some effort should be made to assess pain severity. People with OA report many different patterns of pain: for example, worse with weight-bearing, worse after prolonged sitting, or predominant night pain. Even night pain is complex and may be reported as pain after getting into bed that eases off, pain when the knees bump against each other that wakes the individual, or a deep-seated pain that wakes the individual. The pathological significance of these different pains is unclear, but it may be that different treatments are required. Of course, any history of newly occurring night pain, especially in a young patient, should prompt a search for bony tumors.

Many patients presenting with OA may have had symptoms for a long time. The complexities of chronic pain and its intimate relationship with coping mechanisms and mood are therefore involved. When taking a history, it is worthwhile making some simple assessment of features associated with chronic pain, including sleep disturbance and mood alteration (see *Fast Facts: Chronic and Cancer Pain*).

Assessment of quality of life. Some assessment of functional limitations associated with the particular joint disorder is required. For lower limb problems this may be an assessment of how far the

TABLE 5.1

Presenting features of inflammatory arthritis and osteoarthritis

Inflammatory arthritis	Osteoarthritis
• Prolonged early morning stiffness for 30–60 minutes	• A few minutes of early morning pain and stiffness, with relief from pain and 'freeing up' or loosening of the joint after repeated movement • 'Disuse' pain and stiffness after periods of immobility • General worsening of symptoms at end of the day, after repetitive weight-bearing tasks involving the affected joints or after prolonged walking or standing
• Distribution of joint disease: a symmetric small-joint polyarthritis might suggest rheumatoid arthritis; onset of bilateral shoulder and pelvic girdle pain might suggest polymyalgia rheumatica	• Tends to be asymmetric with one or two joints involved, especially large weight-bearing joints; nodal disease can be symmetric
• Presence of known diseases associated with an inflammatory arthritis (e.g. psoriasis, inflammatory bowel disease) or infections (e.g. sexually transmitted diseases and diarrheal illnesses)	• Previous significant joint injury or previous joint surgery (e.g. meniscectomy)
• Features associated with a connective tissue disease, including photosensitivity, mouth ulcers or rash	• Relevant occupational history of heavy, repetitive loading of joints
• A definite family history of inflammatory arthritis (don't forget gout)	• Often need some caution interpreting responses, as many people are unaware of the different types of arthritis

subject can walk unaided and the degree of difficulty with common activities of daily living such as getting out of chairs, or using toilets, baths and showers. Impact on hobbies such as golf or on ability to care for a relative may be the reason prompting presentation. Importantly, the effect of joint pain on occupation should be noted.

Presence of comorbidities. As mentioned previously, many people with OA of one joint will have pain in other joint areas. The usual OA age group has significant comorbidities, which must be assessed in order to guide therapy appropriately.

Physical examination

General inspection of the individual joint will include observation of gait and looking for previous surgical scars or joint deformity. Examination findings in the OA joint may include:

- tenderness (most marked over the joint line)
- crepitus
- swelling (synovial or bony)
- reduced range of movement
- malalignment.

The following sections highlight important points in the examination of individual joints.

Hands. In the small joints of the hands, findings range from minimal tenderness to marked bony enlargement and deformity, with Heberden's nodes at the distal interphalangeal joint and Bouchard's nodes at the proximal interphalangeal joints (Figure 5.4).

There may be tenderness at the base of the thumb in the anatomic snuffbox, or marked 'squaring' of the base of the thumb. Careful attention should be taken when examining the thumb joints in order to avoid confusion between first metacarpophalangeal and first carpometacarpal arthritis, although they commonly occur together (see location in Figure 5.4).

Note that prolonged hand pain of any cause will result in poor grip strength. This will be associated with weak forearm muscles and often some degree of lateral (and to a lesser extent medial)

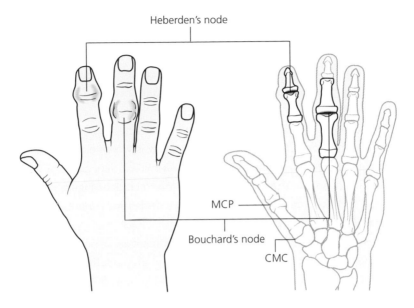

Figure 5.4 Heberden's and Bouchard's nodes in the osteoarthritic hand. Heberden's nodes form in the distal interphalangeal joints, while Bouchard's nodes form in the proximal interphalangeal joints. When examining the thumb, care should be taken to avoid confusion between the first metacarpophalangeal (MCP) joint and the first carpometacarpal (CMC) joint.

epicondylitis, with tenderness over the condylar tendon attachments at the elbow.

Hip. Observation of functional activities, especially walking, will often give a good indication of pain elicited by weight bearing and muscle weakness around the hip joint. Differentiation from lumbar spine problems may be helped by assessing the medial rotation of the hip joint with the patient sitting on a firm surface (the spine and pelvis are therefore supported and relatively fixed in this position, so that any movement elicited by the examiner is likely to be isolated to the hip joint). The symptom of groin pain tends to be specific to the hip joint.

Patients with early OA in the hip normally lose internal rotation first, with later loss of external rotation. Clinical assessment of the hip

53

joint should examine full passive movement of the hip with the patient in a supine position, moving the leg into flexion, then internal rotation and external rotation of the joint with the hip and knee both flexed to 90 degrees (Figure 5.5). Active or passive movement of the hip joint will often reproduce the patient's symptoms and it is important to ask if this is the case.

Knee. During examination of the knee joints it is worth noting varus or valgus deformity (see Figure 4.1, page 41) which may give clues to the site of the major OA compartment involvement (see Figure 2.4, page 24). Malalignment is also a prognostic factor for progression (see Chapter 2) and functional decline.

After palpation for effusions (clinical examination cannot easily distinguish effusions from synovial hypertrophy), palpation of the medial and lateral joint lines often reveals tenderness, bony swelling at the joint margins and overall joint enlargement, which may also be visible.

The presence of a flexion deformity is also useful to note. The joint needs to be moved through the range of flexion to extension to determine the passive range of movement and to detect any

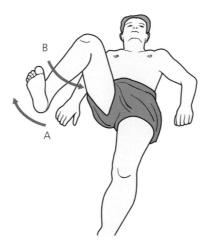

Figure 5.5 Internal (A) and external (B) hip rotation to assess range of motion and extension.

mechanical block to movement. Early in the disease, patients may have a flexion deformity that is reversible with appropriate therapy, while a fixed flexion deformity may imply a poor outcome with conservative therapy.

Tests for medial–lateral laxity should be performed by applying varus and valgus stress to the slightly flexed knee (Figure 5.6a). Likewise, anterior–posterior laxity is assessed by gliding the tibia anteriorly and posteriorly on the femur (Figure 5.6b).

The patella can be moved passively in both lateral–medial and proximal–distal movements, with gentle compression onto the femoral surface to assess for crepitus and pain, which may indicate OA changes in the patellofemoral compartment. Patellofemoral joint pain and crepitus can also be elicited by asking the patient to perform a half-squat.

(a)

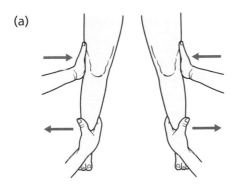

(b)

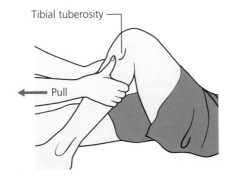

Figure 5.6 (a) Detection of medial and lateral collateral ligament laxity, by stressing the ligaments while the legs are extended and relaxed. (b) Detection of anterior crucial ligament laxity.

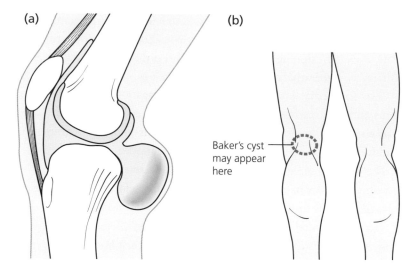

Figure 5.7 When the back of the knee joint becomes swollen, the synovial fluid increases and spills into the bursa in the hollow at the back of the knee, causing it to increase in size and creating a popliteal (Baker's) cyst. (a) Interior view of a Baker's cyst. (b) Location of the cyst at the back of the knee, which can be detected by external palpation.

Palpate for a Baker's (popliteal) cyst (Figure 5.7) – these are quite common in moderate-to-severe OA and reflect OA changes within the knee joint and a knee effusion. They may be asymptomatic or present with:

- a rounded swelling at the back of the knee (can be the size of a golf ball)
- a sensation of pressure in the back of the joint, which can go down into the calf muscle (may indicate rupture of the cyst; the associated acute calf swelling is often confused with a deep venous thrombosis)
- difficulties in completely flexing the joint
- aching and tenderness posterior to the knee after exercise.

Investigations

Radiography. In general, the diagnosis of OA is based on clinical history and examination; findings on conventional radiographs do not usually prompt a change of management in early presentations. Since this disease generally presents with symptoms, these should be addressed first. Radiographs may be helpful if there are diagnostic difficulties at particular sites (see below), or to establish the structural severity of OA. The typical radiographic findings (see Figures 2.5–2.7, page 25) are:

- joint-space narrowing (for the knee, make sure you are looking at films taken when the patient is weight bearing)
- osteophytes
- subchondral bone thickening or sclerosis
- subchondral bone cyst formation
- chondrocalcinosis – calcification of areas of the hyaline cartilage
- small calcified foreign bodies (these are usually of little clinical significance in the absence of true knee locking).

If assessing the severity of knee OA with radiography, it is important to order images taken when the patient is weight bearing, as joint-space narrowing cannot be accurately assessed in images in which the patient is supine. Interestingly, using more than one radiographic view increases the diagnostic yield: a large study demonstrated that a posteroanterior view of the knee showed an OA prevalence of 57% in a cohort of painful knees, while addition of a skyline (axial) or lateral view (used to identify patellofemoral OA) increased this prevalence to 87%.

Blood tests for inflammation (e.g. C-reactive protein [CRP], erythrocyte sedimentation rate [ESR]) may be a useful adjunct in differential diagnosis of mechanical and inflammatory problems, although they are non-specific. Elevations of these markers beyond normal reference ranges (and age and sex corrections for ESR) in patients with prolonged morning stiffness greatly increase the likelihood of an inflammatory arthritis. The rheumatoid factor and antinuclear antibody tests are not good screening tools for RA or systemic lupus erythematosus, respectively, as they have low sensitivity in the normal population. The relatively new anti-citrullinated cyclic peptide (anti-CCP) test has high specificity for later development of RA and its use as a screening test in OA is being evaluated.

Synovial fluid examination for crystals (both calcium and urate) is extremely useful in difficult diagnostic cases. Aspiration of small joints in such cases may be aided by ultrasound guidance. Calcium pyrophosphate crystals may be present even in the absence of a 'pseudogout' presentation.

Modern imaging modalities. Ultrasonography and MRI are more sensitive than clinical examination in detecting synovitis and effusions (and in distinguishing between the two), but the presence of either pathology does not usually differentiate mechanical from inflammatory arthritides. Although MRI has been useful in informing us on the pathology and causes of pain in OA, it has no role in the routine assessment of the OA joint. MRI-detected meniscal tears are not an indication for surgical intervention in the OA knee unless there are clear locking symptoms. Perhaps in the future MRI may be useful for targeting therapies to particular OA subsets.

Differential diagnoses at specific sites

At the hand. The major differential diagnosis for multiple hand small-joint pain and swelling is between RA and OA with secondary inflammation. Generally, the absence of prolonged morning stiffness and the examination findings of bony deformities suggest an OA problem, but rheumatologic opinion may be required. However, pain at the base of the thumb (the first carpometacarpal joint) with local wrist pain can be difficult to distinguish from carpal tunnel syndrome, and sometimes the conditions coexist. Features of pain or parasthesia in the thumb and second and third fingers, together with early morning or night awakening, clinically point to carpal tunnel syndrome. Polyarticular gout can sometimes complicate OA of small joints.

At the shoulder. The commonest cause of shoulder pain in patients over the age of 55 is subacromial impingement syndrome, which includes rotated cuff pathology and/or subacromial bursitis. The next commonest pathology is probably capsulitis, with marked restriction of shoulder movement. Acromioclavicular OA is not uncommon, although the exact frequency is not clear. This may be a difficult diagnosis to make in the presence of generalized shoulder pain with associated functional disability and may require the use of radiographic or ultrasonographic imaging of the acromioclavicular joint. In the person with longstanding rotator cuff pathology or other trauma, true glenohumeral OA may be present.

At the hip. Many patients believe that hip pain occurs on the outer lateral aspect of the thigh and this is commonly what presents as 'hip pain'. However, true hip pain is generally felt in the groin or deep buttock (and may occasionally be referred to the thigh or knee). Patients with true hip disease often have difficulty putting on shoes and socks. Much more commonly, outer thigh pain represents trochanteric bursalgia or bursitis, which has the following features (Figure 5.8):

- pain on the outer aspect of the thigh that is worse when lying on at night or with repeated walking and weight bearing

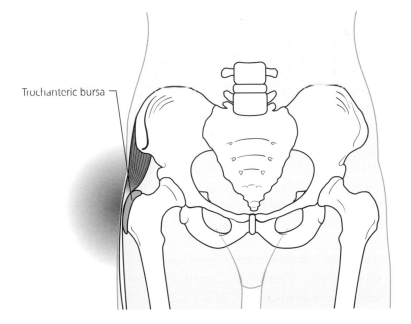

Trochanteric bursa

Figure 5.8 Location of the pain of trochanteric bursitis.

- pain radiating down the outside of the thigh to the knee
- focal tenderness over the trochanteric bursal region.

True hip OA may often have an element of trochanteric bursitis as well. It is common for patients with OA of the knee (or indeed who are limping for any reason) to develop secondary trochanteric bursitis.

At the knee. In the typical older patient with OA, a history of a knee 'giving way' usually reflects quadriceps weakness rather than ligamentous instability or meniscal problem.

True mechanical locking should be distinguished from 'gelling' – in the former, patients will often describe the knee locking in mid-gait and requiring some manipulation to return joint function; in the latter (a much more common symptom), patients report that pain prevents them from bending the knee after prolonged immobility (e.g. after kneeling). This distinction is important, since true locking suggests meniscal pathology or a loose body that may respond to arthroscopic intervention.

As individuals with OA of the knee are also at risk for knee-region pain originating from outside of the joint, it is important to think about periarticular causes of knee pain, such as iliotibial band syndrome or infrapatellar or anserine bursitis (Figure 5.9).

At the foot and ankle. The differential diagnosis of problems with the first metatarsophalangeal joint is most often between OA, a bunion and gout. Often, if attacks of gout have been frequent enough the two problems may coexist and it is often difficult to determine if 'gouty' arthritis is still playing a role. Again, any history suggesting inflammatory arthritis, such as prolonged early morning stiffness, may suggest a persistent element of gouty arthritis, whereas a few minutes of morning stiffness but prolonged pain with weight bearing suggests OA. Aspiration of the first metatarsophalangeal or ankle joints is possible using a fine-gauge needle, and has been made easier with the use of ultrasound. Pragmatically, a trial of urate-lowering therapy may sometimes be required.

One of the biggest problems with forefoot diagnoses is the co-presentation of different problems. Bunions may coexist with OA of

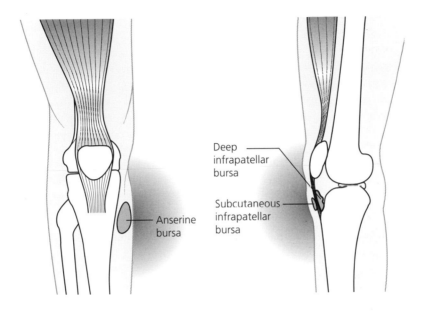

Figure 5.9 Sites of knee bursitis.

the first metatarsophalangeal joint, and intermetatarsal head bursitis (especially with weight-bearing pain between the first and second, and second and third metatarsal heads) is also common. True ankle joint OA (i.e. at the tibiotalar joint with reduced plantar and dorsiflexion) is uncommon without a preceding history of trauma. A radiograph of the ankle may be useful to make a definitive diagnosis in such cases.

Key points – diagnosis

- Careful history taken together with clinical examination of joints establishes most diagnoses.
- Radiographic and laboratory investigations may occasionally aid the assessment process.
- Differential diagnosis from other rheumatologic conditions and inflammatory arthritides is part of the diagnostic process.

Key references

Bijlsma JW, Berenbaum F, Lafeber FP. Osteoarthritis: an update with relevance for clinical practice. *Lancet* 2011;377:2115–26.

Cousins MJ, Gallagher RM. *Fast Facts: Chronic and Cancer Pain*, 2nd edn. Oxford: Health Press Limited, 2011.

Duncan RC, Hay EM, Saklatvala J, Croft PR. Prevalence of radiographic osteoarthritis – it all depends on your point of view. *Rheumatology* 2006;45:757–60.

Peat G, Thomas E, Duncan R et al. Clinical classification criteria for knee osteoarthritis: performance in the general population and primary care. *Ann Rheum Dis* 2006;65:1363–7.

Prevention versus treatment

Current therapy of osteoarthritis (OA) largely aims to treat existing disease by controlling its major symptom – pain – and maintain or improve joint and limb function and improve quality of life. While there are numerous therapies targeted against symptoms, at present no treatments have been definitively shown to modify the structural progression of OA.

Currently, the best advice we can give on preventing OA relates to the following lifestyle modifications:

- avoid joint trauma
- avoid high-impact loading of joints (through sport or occupation)
- maintain a body mass index (BMI) within the normal range for size
- maintain aerobic fitness, which aids periarticular muscle strength and weight control.

A healthy diet is important to aid weight control, but no diets or dietary supplements have been shown to prevent, or to modify the progression of, OA.

Management of OA

The large number of evidence-based guidelines for managing OA agree on several main principles for the treatment of the disease.

- People with OA should be involved in their own management, and should receive education about their condition and the range and safety of treatment options available.
- Optimum treatment involves a combination of non-pharmacological and pharmacological approaches, starting with those therapies with moderate efficacy and low potential toxicity such as exercise, weight loss and paracetamol (acetaminophen).
- Therapies need to be tailored according to an individual person's comorbidities and risk factors.

The Osteoarthritis Research Society International has performed a critical review of the many available guidelines for OA and reported

63

the therapies on which these guidelines commonly agreed (Table 6.1). In practice, many patients will need to try multiple therapies, including non-pharmacological and drug therapies. Generally, the safest effective therapies are recommended as first line – for example, the UK guidelines produced by the National Institute for Health and Clinical Excellence (NICE) recommend 'core' and adjunctive therapies (Figure 6.1).

Very importantly, we should not confuse what clinicians advise or prescribe with how patients manage their own OA. There is little research on what patients actually do, but certainly compliance,

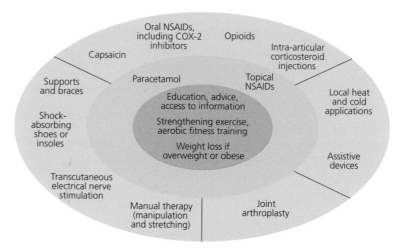

Figure 6.1 Treatments for osteoarthritis (OA) in adults. Starting at the center and working outward, the treatments are arranged in the order in which they should be considered, taking into account individuals' different needs, risk factors and preferences. The core treatments (in the center) should be considered first for every person with OA. If further treatment is required, the drugs in the second circle should be considered before those in the outer circle. The outer circle also shows adjunctive treatments (both non-pharmacological and surgical), which have less well-proved efficacy, provide less symptom relief or confer an increased risk to the patient than those in the second circle. Reproduced from Conaghan et al. 2008 with permission from BMJ Publishing Group Ltd.

TABLE 6.1

Effect size (ES) for selected non-surgical modalities with Ia level of evidence and significant effect, for treatment of knee and hip OA (for both unless otherwise noted)

Modality	ES for pain (95% CI)
Non-pharmacological	
Self-management	0.06 (0.02, 0.10)
Telephone	0.12 (0.00, 0.24)
Education	0.06 (0.03, 0.10)
Strengthening	Knee: 0.32 (0.23, 0.42)
	Hip: 0.38 (0.08, 0.68)
Aerobic exercise	Knee: 0.52 (0.34, 0.70)
Water-based exercise	0.19 (0.04, 0.35)
Weight reduction	Knee: 0.20 (0.00, 0.39)
Acupuncture	Knee: 0.35 (0.15, 0.55), *0.22 (0.01, 0.44)
Pharmacological	
Paracetamol (acetaminophen)	0.14 (0.05, 0.23), *0.10 (−0.03, 0.23)
NSAIDs	0.29 (0.22, 0.35), *0.39 (0.24, 0.55)
COX-2 inhibitors	0.44 (0.33, 0.55)
Topical NSAIDs	Knee: 0.44 (0.27, 0.62), *0.42 (0.19, 0.65)
Opioids	0.78 (0.59, 0.98)
Intra-articular corticosteroid	Knee: 0.58 (0.34, 0.75)
Intra-articular hyaluronans	Knee: 0.60 (0.37, 0.83), *0.22 (−0.11, 0.54)
Glucosamine sulfate	0.58 (0.30, 0.87), *0.29 (0.0003, 0.57)
Chondroitin sulfate	0.75 (0.50, 1.01), *0.0005 (−0.11, 0.12)
Avocado soybean unsaponifiables	0.38 (0.01, 0.76)
Rosehip	0.37 (0.13, 0.60)

CI, confidence interval; COX, cyclooxygenase; ES, effect size; NSAID, non-steroidal anti-inflammatory drug; OA, osteoarthritis.
ES of 0.2 is considered small; 0.5 is moderate; > 0.8 is large.
Ia level of evidence is from meta-analysis of randomized controlled trials.
*ES when analysis limited to high-quality trials.
Adapted from Zhang et al. 2010.

perhaps more so with exercise therapies, is often low. Clinicians therefore need to adapt the consultation to the needs of the individual patient to reach agreement on a suitable management plan.

The subsequent chapters give an overview of the rationale, evidence and clinical hints for using a particular therapy. However, it is worth first reviewing some of the limitations of the evidence base.

Problems with interpreting the OA therapy literature

The practicing clinician may well be overwhelmed at times with the number of publications on a given therapy. However, some critical analysis of trial data is important. Some of the common problems in interpreting OA trials include:

- the use of different definitions (e.g. of OA)
- the absence of a patient-relevant outcome
- unrealistic inclusion criteria
- the degree of clinical significance.

Different definitions. Studies use different definitions of OA, focusing on symptoms, radiographic findings, or a combination of both. Inclusion of a wide range of pain severity (and presumably a wide range of structural pathology) means that the effects of a therapy on subgroups may be missed. Many studies of knee OA do not evaluate the patellofemoral joint, which is a common site of pain in OA of the knee.

Absence of a patient-relevant outcome. Commonly, studies use a pain visual analog scale, and recent studies include multidomain instruments such as the Western Ontario MacMaster questionnaire (commonly known as WOMAC), which is a patient-completed form with questions on pain, stiffness and function. However, is pain the only relevant outcome we should be studying? Modern trial guidelines recommend assessing other domains that are relevant to people with OA. These might include depression, sleep scales, patient global assessments and specifically developed quality-of-life assessment tools. Such information should be gathered in addition to instruments evaluating pain and function.

Non-generalizable inclusion criteria. Most trials (of drugs in particular) tend to include relatively healthy patients and do not reflect the usual older OA population with a high frequency of comorbidities. In addition, trial participants may have only one painful joint, whereas large community samples suggest that, in practice, patients over 55 years of age may have an average of four painful joints.

Degree of clinical significance. Many studies have reported a statistically significant difference between two trial therapies without reporting whether the result is important clinically. This may sometimes be expressed as the minimal clinically important difference (MCID). The MCID may vary depending on the measure used to estimate a patient's symptoms. Although the reader should look at specific data for individual outcome measures, in general, a treatment effect of at least 20% is desirable.

Key points – principles of management

- Prevention currently means advice to avoid trauma and high-impact repetitive loading of joints.
- Essential management requires involving and educating the person and choosing a range of non-pharmacological and pharmacological therapies.
- Safe therapies with low toxicity and good efficacy, such as muscle strengthening, aerobic exercise and paracetamol (acetaminophen), are a good starting point for management.

Key references

American College of Rheumatology Subcommittee on Osteoarthritis Guidelines. Special article: recommendations for the medical management of osteoarthritis of the hip and knee. *Arthritis Rheum* 2000;43:1905–15.

Conaghan PG, Dickson J, Grant RL. Care and management of osteoarthritis in adults: summary of NICE guidance. *BMJ* 2008;336: 502–3.

Jordan KM, Arden NK, Doherty M et al. EULAR Recommendations 2003: an evidence based approach to the management of knee osteoarthritis: report of a task force of the Standing Committee for International Clinical Studies Including Therapeutic Trials (ESCISIT). *Ann Rheum Dis* 2003;62: 1145–55.

Zhang W, Doherty M, Arden N et al. EULAR evidence based recommendations for the management of hip osteoarthritis: report of a task force for the EULAR Standing Committee for International Clinical Studies Including Therapeutics (ESCISIT). *Ann Rheum Dis* 2005;64:669–81.

Zhang W, Doherty M, Leeb BF et al. EULAR evidence based recommendations for the management of hand osteoarthritis: report of a task force for the EULAR Standing Committee for International Clinical Studies Including Therapeutics (ESCISIT). *Ann Rheum Dis* 2007;66:377–88.

Zhang W, Moskowitz RW, Nuki G et al. OARSI recommendations for the management of hip and knee osteoarthritis. Part I: Critical appraisal of existing treatment guidelines and systematic review of current research evidence. *Osteoarthritis Cartilage* 2007;15:981–1000.

Zhang W, Moskowitz RW, Nuki G et al. OARSI recommendations for the management of hip and knee osteoarthritis. Part II: OARSI evidence-based, expert consensus guidelines. *Osteoarthritis Cartilage* 2008;16:137–62.

Zhang W, Nuki G, Moskowitz RW et al. OARSI recommendations for the management of hip and knee osteoarthritis: part III: changes in evidence following systematic cumulative update of research published through January 2009. *Osteoarthritis Cartilage* 2010; 18:476–99.

7

Non-pharmacological management

The aim of this chapter is to provide a brief overview of the non-pharmacological therapies listed in Chapter 6 (see Figure 6.1, page 64).

Education

Providing patients with information about osteoarthritis (OA) and its treatment is an essential first step. Rheumatology societies in most countries provide easy-to-read brochures or booklets on OA that can be given to patients at consultations. Major sites on the Internet may also be a useful source of information, such as the Arthritis Care and Arthritis Research Campaign websites in the UK, and the Arthritis Foundation website in the USA (see Useful resources, pages 108–9).

Several studies suggest that patient education is a valuable adjunctive therapy in OA, although by itself the effects on pain are relatively small; effects on other important drivers of quality of life such as self-efficacy (the belief that one has the ability to successfully perform a specific behavior to achieve an outcome) may be more substantial. Some data suggest that both individualized education strategies and group education may improve patient symptoms.

Self-management

Education and exercise are components of a self-management program, but other issues such as spousal/partner support, emotional aspects and coping skills, such as relaxation and distraction methods, can also be addressed. An understanding of appropriate activity and rest cycles may improve adherence to exercise programs, while dietary modifications can encourage weight loss, contributing to the overall success of a program. As might be expected, these programs have small effect sizes on physical outcomes, but moderate effects on psychosocial outcomes in OA.

Exercise

The benefits of exercise may be mediated through different routes, including increased strength and endurance, weight reduction, more accurate proprioception and joint position sense, improvement in comorbidities and reduction in anxiety or depression. Numerous studies have examined the benefits of exercise for OA of the knee and a few studies have assessed the benefits of exercise for OA of the hip. On balance, these studies show that therapeutic exercise brings about a moderate reduction in pain and some improvement in function, although the nature of the exercise differs between studies. It appears that benefits arise from individual programs, group classes and for exercises performed at home. Not surprisingly, the benefits of exercise may not be sustained for more than a few months if the exercises are not continued; it is therefore important to consider not only patient adherence but also the longer-term use of strategies such as an intermittent overview by a physical therapist to encourage ongoing exercise. Organizations such as the Arthritis Foundation in the USA and Arthritis Care in the UK (see Useful resources, pages 108–9) provide a range of individual and group programs geared toward people with OA.

Exercise for OA patients may take two forms:

- strengthening local muscles (e.g. quadriceps for OA of the knee)
- aerobic training.

Strengthening exercises. Patients may not be able to undertake aerobic fitness training until they have sufficiently strengthened local muscles. It is worth considering that walking on a leg with very weak quadriceps muscles may in fact aggravate symptoms, leading to falls, without producing much benefit.

A range of effective exercises are available to help reduce OA knee symptoms, including both strengthening exercises and aerobic walking. Such exercises should be tailored to the individual.

One simple exercise for quadriceps strengthening is demonstrated in Figure 7.1. The patient lies on a flat surface and bends up the non-exercising leg (to take some strain off the lower back and hips). The knee to be exercised is extended fully and pushed down towards the bed or supporting surface. The patient can be asked to pull their toes back at the same time, which adds a hamstring stretch to this exercise. With the knee fully extended the patient then lifts the leg for

(a)

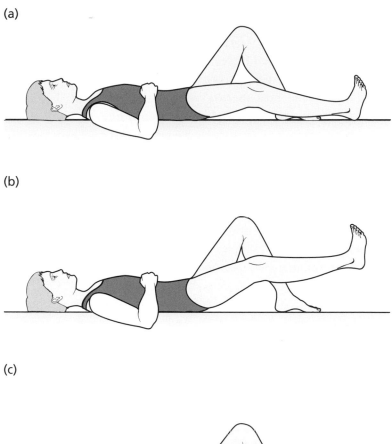

(b)

(c)

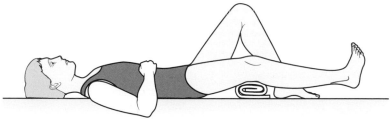

Figure 7.1 (a,b) Exercise for strengthening the quadriceps muscle in patients with osteoarthritis of the knee (see text for details). (c) Patients with a weak quadriceps muscle should start with an 'inner-range' quadriceps exercise using a rolled-up towel placed under the affected knee. The knee should be pushed down to fully extend it into the towel, while simultaneously lifting the heel off the bed.

a count of 10–20 seconds. Multiple repetitions on both sides are encouraged. However, not uncommonly, a patient may not be able to do this straight-leg raise off the bed, in which case it may be useful to start with an 'inner-range' quadriceps exercise using a rolled-up towel placed directly under the affected knee. Pushing down with the knee to fully extend it into the towel and simultaneously lifting the heel off the bed provides an easier way of doing the straight-leg raise exercise.

For patients who are this weak, another helpful exercise may be walking laps in a swimming pool. This exercise may also be helpful for hip pain (due to true hip OA or trochanteric bursitis), where weak quadriceps will contribute to abnormal biomechanical load.

A lateral leg raise may also be helpful in hip problems. Here the person lies on their side and lifts the leg to be exercised towards the ceiling for a count of 10–20 seconds (Figure 7.2).

Aerobic exercise is associated with improvement in well being and level of conditioning, both of which are key determinants of physical function and disability in OA.

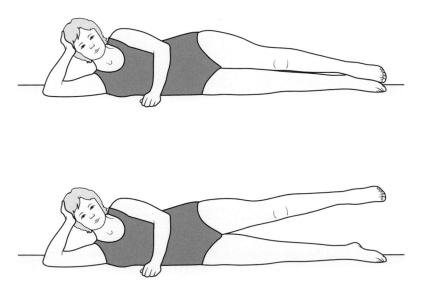

Figure 7.2 Lateral leg raise for patients with osteoarthritis of the hips.

Once a person has strong enough quadriceps (see above), options for aerobic exercise include:

- walking laps in a swimming pool
- swimming
- cycling on an exercise bike, although this may be limited by the degree of patellofemoral disease
- use of cross-trainer or glider machines; patients who are getting stronger must be careful not to undertake gymnasium activities using machines that put untoward force through the knee or hip (e.g. 'stepper'-type machines)
- walking – if it can be done at a reasonable pace
- cycling on the road.

In individuals with anatomic deformity (e.g. knee malalignment), it is wise to initiate strengthening/resistance exercise programs with training by a physical therapist.

Weight loss

This is a hugely important area given the obesity epidemic facing Western societies, with its attendant risk for both incidence and progression of OA. Although there appears to be great face validity in the concept of reducing mechanical force through a large joint by weight reduction, only a few randomized trials have examined the efficacy of this therapy. Recent work suggests that the combination of dietary weight loss and an exercise class can result in significant long-term reduction of pain and improvement in physical function in patients who are overweight. This finding is probably not surprising given that dietary change alone is often not sufficient to produce effective weight loss; the major problem faced by people with OA is trying to find an exercise program that is suitable when they already have one or more painful joints. Dietary change needs more than just 'you need to lose weight'; expert advice including education on food nutritional value is part of an effective diet program.

Devices

Again, although there appears good face validity for using mechanical devices to 'unload' a joint, there is a paucity of good trial evidence to support these therapies. A walking stick is certainly useful in preventing falls, but should be used in combination with appropriate strengthening exercises. Evidence suggests that high-heeled shoes may increase medial compartment forces in the knee during walking. Recent work suggests that barefoot mechanics (achieved through barefoot or thin-soled walking shoes) may improve joint loads in OA while thick, 'supportive' shoes may actually increase such loads, though the effects on OA symptoms at the knee or the foot have not been well investigated.

Only a few studies have examined valgus bracing in medial knee OA (with a varus deformity). At present there is insufficient evidence from long-term randomized trials with appropriate control groups to support the use of this modality. Similarly, there is conflicting evidence regarding the usefulness of insoles for reducing knee pain, such as the lateral wedge insole for medial tibiofemoral OA.

Patella taping for predominant patellofemoral joint OA has been useful in some short-term clinical studies, but compliance is unknown and the technique has to be taught by an expert. A thumb splint may be useful in patients who have OA at the base of the thumb.

Electrotherapies

Transcutaneous electrical nerve stimulation (TENS), which involves pulsed, alternating-frequency electrical stimulation, has been popular for the management of chronic pain for some years. Previous evidence of potential benefit of TENS in knee OA was not confirmed in a systematic review, although large, high-quality trials were lacking. A few good studies have demonstrated convincing beneficial effects for other modalities such as laser pulsed electromagnetic field and ultrasound therapies in OA of the knee, but there are very few data on OA in other sites.

Acupuncture

Acupuncture has gained increasing popularity amongst patients and clinicians in Western countries. It is applied in a variety of ways, either using traditional Chinese techniques (including addition of herbs) or westernized approaches. Sometimes electrical stimulation is added (electroacupuncture). Complex neurophysiological mechanisms have been suggested in an attempt to explain its mechanism of action, which may be partially mediated through patient–provider interactions. While some meta-analyses of trials in this area have demonstrated positive benefits, others have not. Further understanding of the role of acupuncture, and in particular the subgroups that might benefit, seems worthwhile.

Complementary medicines

It is well documented that individuals with OA use large amounts of complementary (often over-the-counter) medications, with up to 40% of subjects reporting use in some studies. These supplements include cod liver oil, evening primrose oil, and celery and garlic extracts. No good clinical trial evidence exists to support the use of these therapies for OA, and little is known of their potential toxicity. A major issue for all these medicines is quality control, particularly as many patients order these preparations from 'off-shore' companies.

Glucosamine and chondroitin sulfate. It has been suggested, on the basis of conventional radiographic studies, that both of these oral agents act as structure-modifying drugs in people with OA of the knee, reducing the rate of cartilage loss. While such findings are based on small numbers of studies, these agents certainly have minimal reported side effects. There remains significant controversy regarding the role of these medications in OA management.

Glucosamine is a component of the glycosaminoglycans that make up articular cartilage (see Chapter 1, pages 9–11). Oral glucosamine (produced synthetically or from shellfish shells) is well absorbed, but there are no convincing data in humans to suggest it reaches the joint. Twenty randomized controlled trials have compared glucosamine with placebo in patients with OA of the knee and/or hip. A recent meta-analysis of these studies suggests a moderate reduction in pain for users of glucosamine sulfate, 1500 mg/day, but not of glucosamine hydrochloride; the effect size was small (effect size 0.29, 95% confidence interval [CI] 0.0003, 0.57) when limited to high-quality studies only. No substantial structure modification effect has been reproducibly shown. It may take a few months for the effects to be evident, so it is not a good alternative to a short-term analgesic.

Chondroitin sulfate is another glycosaminoglycan component of the extracellular matrix of cartilage and is also found in the extracellular matrix of bone, skin and tendons. Synthesized chondroitin is available as an oral agent, sometimes in combination with glucosamine. Again, it is not clear how this oral agent may directly affect the joint. A recent meta-analysis of 20 trials demonstrated a moderate to large effect size (0.75, 95% CI 0.50, 0.99), but when restricted to high-quality trials this became insignificant (effect size 0.0005, 95% CI –0.11, 0.12). There is a suggestion of small reductions in the rate of decline of joint space width in four industry-sponsored trials of chondroitin sulfate, with an effect size of 0.26 (95% CI 0.16, 0.36).

Diet and dietary supplements

Despite many myths about the effects of diet on joints, there is no good evidence for any effects beyond those mediated by obesity. Epidemiological data suggest that low dietary intake of vitamin D and low serum 25-hydroxyvitamin D_3 levels have been associated with radiological progression of knee OA. However, a 2-year double-blind placebo-controlled clinical trial for symptomatic knee OA found no benefit from vitamin D_3 (target serum level > 30 ng/mL) for a variety of outcomes (WOMAC score [see page 66], physical function, cartilage volume loss by MRI, or minimum joint space width on radiographs).

A well-designed trial showed that vitamin E supplements were ineffective in relieving OA symptoms in the knee.

Key points – non-pharmacological management

- Education, self-management and exercise are important components of treatment.
- Muscle strengthening if weak and then aerobic exercises are the key to good management.
- Use of proper footwear, and weight reduction in overweight individuals, will reduce biomechanical loading of joints and improve symptoms.
- Use of aids such as a walking stick or devices to aid everyday activities (e.g. for opening jars) can also help symptoms and improve participation.
- The effects of many non-pharmacological therapies are difficult to discern because of differences in study designs and heterogeneous outcomes.

Key references

Brouwer RW, van Raaij TM, Jakma TS et al. Braces and orthoses for treating osteoarthritis of the knee. *Cochrane Database Syst Rev* 2005;1:CD004020.

Christensen R, Bartels EM, Astrup A, Bliddal H. Effect of weight reduction in obese patients diagnosed with knee osteoarthritis: a systematic review and meta-analysis. *Ann Rheum Dis* 2007;66:433–9.

Devos-Comby L, Cronan T, Roesch SC. Do exercise and self-management interventions benefit patients with osteoarthritis of the knee? A metaanalytic review. *J Rheumatol* 2006;33:744–56.

Manheimer E, Linde K, Lao L et al. Meta-analysis: acupuncture for osteoarthritis of the knee. *Ann Intern Med* 2007;146:868–77.

McAlindon TE, Dawson-Hughes B, Driban J et al. Clinical trial of vitamin D to reduce pain and structural progression of knee osteoarthritis (OA). *Arthritis Rheum* 2010;62(suppl 10):706abstr.

Reichenbach S, Sterchi R, Scherer M et al. Meta-analysis: chondroitin for osteoarthritis of the knee or hip. *Ann Intern Med* 2007;146:580–90.

Roddy E, Zhang W, Doherty M. Aerobic walking or strengthening exercise for osteoarthritis of the knee? A systematic review. *Ann Rheum Dis* 2005;64:544–8.

Rutjes AW, Nuesch E, Sterchi R et al. Transcutaneous electrical nerve stimulation for osteoarthritis of the knee. *Cochrane Database Syst Rev* 2009;4:CD002823.

Shakoor N, Sengupta M, Foucher KC et al. Effects of common footwear on joint loading in osteoarthritis of the knee. *Arthritis Care Res* 2010;62:917–23.

Vlad SC, LaValley MP, McAlindon TE, Felson DT. Glucosamine for pain in osteoarthritis. Why do trial results differ? *Arthritis Rheum* 2007;56:2267–77.

8

Pharmacological management

This chapter provides an overview of the pharmacological therapies listed in Chapter 6 (see Figure 6.1, page 64) and their potential side effects. As mentioned previously, these therapies largely manage the pain of OA.

It is worth considering the optimal timing of analgesia, that is, when the patient has most symptoms (see page 89). Furthermore, the management of any chronic musculoskeletal pain should always prompt evaluation – and occasionally pharmacological management of – associated sleep and mood disorders.

Therapies with a good safety profile

Paracetamol (acetaminophen) is a well-tolerated first-line analgesic for OA. The site of action of the drug, which has some weak anti-inflammatory action, seems to be in the central nervous system (CNS). Paracetamol is generally safe in doses up to 3–4 g/day and may be effective at lower doses; many people do not take adequate regular doses, probably because they are concerned about the number of tablets required. Paracetamol can also be used in combination with oral agents such as non-steroidal anti-inflammatory drugs (NSAIDs) or in formulations with mild opioids.

Side effects. Paracetamol is metabolized by the liver and can accumulate in patients with chronic liver disease. The major concern lies in overdose, which can lead to acute hepatic toxicity that may be enhanced by alcohol. Despite its relative safety, recent data suggest that high-dose paracetamol (4 g/day) may still lead to upper gastrointestinal side effects, including bleeding, and may negatively affect renal function and blood pressure with daily use.

Topical NSAIDs have been shown to relieve symptoms in OA of the knee and hand. Multiple daily applications (2–4 times a day depending on the product) are usually required, which may limit compliance.

Side effects. NSAIDs are generally very well tolerated. The commonest problems with topical NSAIDs are burning, itch and rash at the site of application. Low systemic levels of absorbed NSAID mean much less gastrointestinal (GI) toxicity than with oral NSAIDs.

Topical capsaicin is derived from hot chili peppers. The strength of the preparations generally used in OA trials is 0.025%, and usually three or four applications a day are required. A small number of randomized controlled trials in OA involving various peripheral joints have demonstrated a small effect in reducing symptoms.

Side effects. The commonest problem is burning of the skin in the area of application, which may subside after 1–2 weeks of continuous use.

Therapies with significant side effects
NSAIDs and COX-2 selective inhibitors

NSAIDs are used by almost 50% of people with OA, although little is known about patterns of long-term usage. The data on use are further complicated by the availability of over-the-counter NSAIDs.

NSAIDs probably work by preventing formation of prostaglandin derivatives by inhibiting the cyclooxygenase (COX)-1 and -2 enzymes. The COX-1 enzyme is thought to be responsible for a constitutive or 'housekeeping' role in important homeostatic functions, such as maintaining gastric mucosal integrity. The COX-2 enzyme is rapidly and substantially induced at sites of inflammation and in some bowel cancers, although it probably also has physiological roles, for example in the kidney. Importantly, as well as being anti-inflammatory agents that work at peripheral sites (rather than in the CNS), NSAIDs are analgesics. Some of the commonly used traditional NSAIDs are ibuprofen, naproxen and diclofenac.

NSAIDs may be more efficacious than paracetamol in certain individuals with OA, although clinical selection of these people on the basis of 'inflammatory' features (such as effusion) is not a good predictor of treatment response. This is not surprising as large studies of OA joints using modern imaging (ultrasound and MRI) have shown that clinical examination is relatively insensitive to the presence of effusions or synovial hypertrophy. A large number of clinical trials of NSAIDs in OA, again predominantly in OA of the knee, have been conducted, mostly of short duration (typically up to 6 weeks). On balance, these studies show moderate reduction in patient symptoms while the NSAID is being used.

COX-2 inhibitors. Drugs with higher COX-2 selectivity (e.g. celecoxib, etoricoxib) were developed in an attempt to reduce the GI toxicity of NSAIDs. Studies have shown that the short-term efficacy of COX-2 inhibitors in OA is similar to that of the traditional NSAIDs. Initial endoscopy studies and subsequent clinical trials have generally supported the concept that COX-2 inhibitors are associated with fewer upper GI problems, including ulceration and serious complications.

Side effects. The widespread use of NSAIDs means that significant morbidity and mortality due to these agents are encountered across communities. The side effects of these commonly used agents will be well known to most readers and are highlighted in Table 8.1.

TABLE 8.1

Side effects of non-steroidal anti-inflammatory drugs

Gastrointestinal

- Dyspepsia
- Gastric erosions
- Peptic ulceration
- Complication of peptic ulcers
- Raised hepatic transaminases

Renal

- Reversible reduction in glomerular filtration rate
- Hyperkalemia
- Interstitial nephritis
- Chronic renal failure

Cardiovascular

- Exacerbation of hypertension and cardiac failure
- Thrombotic cardiovascular events

Central nervous system

- Headache
- Drowsiness
- Confusion

Until recently, GI toxicity was the major recognized side effect for most patients, with approximately a quarter of patients experiencing dyspepsia, diarrhea or abdominal pain; more serious complications (e.g. perforations, ulcers, bleeds) are uncommon. Apart from GI toxicity, COX-2 inhibitors were initially found to have similar side effects to traditional NSAIDs (e.g. raised blood pressure, peripheral edema), but subsequent studies revealed an increased incidence of thrombotic cardiovascular (CV) events. Subsequent analyses now suggest that this increased CV risk is also present with traditional NSAIDs (although the data for naproxen are not as clear). A dose effect may also be present. This has moved to a change in paradigm where it is recognized that COX-2 selectivity by itself does not define the CV risk of these drugs – indeed, traditional NSAIDs and COX-2 inhibitors are increasingly seen as a class of anti-inflammatory agents with a range of side effects (Figure 8.1).

How should NSAIDs and COX-2 inhibitors be prescribed? It is difficult to be didactic, as prescribers must evaluate individual patient risk factors, especially considering the balance of GI and CV risks, and also relevant national guidelines. It is important to remember that these drugs will often be used by older patients with significant comorbidities, who use multiple medications. In general, extra caution should be exercised when using these drugs in elderly patients, as there are higher incidences of important side effects, including confusion. Certainly patients should be fully informed of the potential risks associated with these agents. Table 8.2 provides a summary of prescribing advice with respect to GI and CV risk.

A safe rule is to use the lowest possible dose of drug for the shortest period of time. In the USA, certain insurers/reimbursers require evidence of prior use of the less expensive non-selective NSAIDs before providing prescription coverage for the COX-2-selective NSAIDs.

In the UK, the National Institute for Health and Clinical Excellence (NICE) has recently recommended the routine addition of a proton pump inhibitor (PPI) to either a traditional NSAID or COX-2 inhibitor to reduce the risk of GI side effects. It should be noted, however, that such recommendations were made on the basis of cost-effectiveness for generic, not brand-name, PPIs.

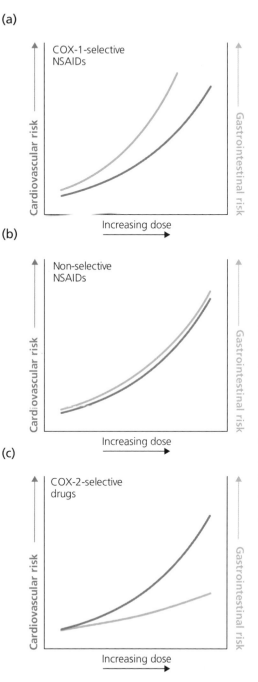

Figure 8.1 Association between dose, cardiovascular risk and gastrointestinal risk for (a) COX-1 selective NSAIDs, (b) non-selective NSAIDs and (c) COX-2 selective drugs. COX, cyclooxygenase; NSAID, non-steroidal anti-inflammatory drug. Reproduced with permission of Elsevier. All rights reserved. Copyright © 2008. From Warner and Mitchell 2008.

TABLE 8.2

Patients in whom prescribing of traditional NSAIDs/COX-2 inhibitors is not recommended

With respect to GI risk, traditional NSAIDs should not be considered in patients:	With respect to CV risk, traditional NSAIDs/COX-2 inhibitors should not be considered in patients:
• over 65 years of age • with a history of peptic ulceration • with a history of GI bleeding or perforation • receiving concomitant medication (e.g. corticosteroids)	• with established ischemic heart disease • with a previous history of stroke • receiving concomitant medication (e.g. ASA [aspirin]) – see text

COX, cyclooxygenase; CV, cardiovascular; GI, gastrointestinal; NSAID, non-steroidal anti-inflammatory drug.

The use of concomitant acetylsalicylic acid (ASA; aspirin) should prompt careful thought about the decision to use an NSAID or COX-2 inhibitor. If a person is using ASA for modest CV risk, then most NSAIDs and COX-2 inhibitors are contraindicated. If GI toxicity is the concern, the GI advantage of a COX-2 inhibitor may be lost after it is combined with ASA. As well, some traditional NSAIDs may interfere with the antiplatelet effect of aspirin.

It is worth monitoring blood pressure and occasionally renal function in people using NSAIDs or COX-2 inhibitors in the long term. In addition, risk factors change over time so periodic review of prescribing is important.

Opioids. All opioids work by acting on endogenous opioid receptors, although specific agents may work at different receptor subtypes. Opioids have been classified as 'weak' or 'strong' but there is some confusion arising from these terms: for example, codeine (often considered a weak opioid) is metabolized to morphine, while many strong opioids are available in low-dose formulations. It is probably more appropriate to consider the dose of an individual agent. Opioids such as codeine, oxycodone and tramadol have been used for many years for the treatment of moderate-to-severe musculoskeletal pain, although there are still relatively few trials in OA. Opioids are recommended in all modern evidence-based OA guidelines, and a meta-analysis of randomized controlled trials demonstrated a benefit of opioids in reducing OA pain, with possibly a lesser effect on improving function.

These drugs may be used in formulations together with paracetamol or ASA. Oxycodone and tramadol are available in slow-release formulations, which may be useful for night pain. Certain therapies, including fentanyl and buprenorphine, are available in transdermal preparations, with some trial data supporting their use in the symptomatic management of OA. These provide sustained release of drug, which may help with compliance in some people.

Side effects. The use of opioids always requires careful consideration of the patient's age, general state, comorbidities and other medications. Common problems include drowsiness and constipation, and rates of withdrawal because of side effects are high in clinical trials and probably in clinical practice. Sometimes tolerance to the drowsiness and CNS-depressant effects will occur within a few days of commencing therapy, but confusion can be a particular problem in the elderly and can contribute to elevated risk of falls. As with all analgesic therapies, it is sensible to start with a low dose and increase as dictated by analgesic efficacy and side effects.

Duloxetine. Previously approved for fibromyalgia, duloxetine was approved in the USA in 2010 for use in chronic musculoskeletal pain, including chronic back pain and pain due to osteoarthritis. Duloxetine is a selective serotonin and norepinephrine reuptake inhibitor that is thought to inhibit centrally mediated pain pathways. Side effects include nausea, insomnia, dizziness, dry mouth, somnolence, constipation and fatigue. Potential hepatotoxicity means that laboratory monitoring is recommended.

Timing of pharmacological interventions

It is worth considering the likely duration of effect of a pharmacological intervention, especially in people who only use analgesics intermittently. For many people with OA, symptoms are worse in the latter half of the day, and taking a short-acting agent such as paracetamol or ibuprofen at lunchtime and/or at evening-meal time may provide maximal short-term benefits. Short-acting agents may also be useful before undertaking a weight-bearing activity that predictably brings on pain, such as going shopping.

When people have symptoms predominantly at night, an agent with a longer half-life may be appropriate to prevent waking. The use of stronger analgesics that cause drowsiness as a side effect may be acceptable as nocturnal medications.

Key points – pharmacological management

- Paracetamol (acetaminophen), topical non-steroidal anti-inflammatory drugs (NSAIDs) and capsaicin are well-tolerated early pharmacological interventions.
- Traditional NSAIDs and cyclooxygenase (COX)-2 inhibitors are effective but have a range of important side effects that must be taken into consideration, including gastrointestinal and cardiovascular risks.
- Care should be taken with titrating the dose of opioids and considering which formulation to use.
- Optimal timing of analgesia should be considered in relation to when the patient has most symptoms and the likely duration of effect of the pharmacological intervention.

Key references

Avouac J, Gossec L, Dougados M. Efficacy and safety of opioids for osteoarthritis: a meta-analysis of randomized controlled trials. *Osteoarthritis Cartilage* 2007; 15:957–65.

Kearney PM, Baigent C, Godwin J et al. Do selective cyclo-oxygenase-2 inhibitors and traditional non-steroidal anti-inflammatory drugs increase the risk of atherothrombosis? Meta-analysis of randomised trials. *BMJ* 2006;332: 1302–8.

McGettigan P, Henry D. Cardiovascular risk and inhibition of cyclooxygenase: a systematic review of the observational studies of selective and nonselective inhibitors of cyclooxygenase 2. *JAMA* 2006;296:1633–44.

Nuesch E, Rutjes AW, Husni E et al. Oral or transdermal opioids for osteoarthritis of the knee or hip. *Cochrane Database Syst Rev* 2009;4:CD003115.

Underwood M, Ashby D, Cross P et al. Advice to use topical or oral ibuprofen for chronic knee pain in older people: randomised controlled trial and patient preference study. *BMJ* 2008;336:138–42.

Warner TD, Mitchell JA. COX-2 selectivity alone does not define the cardiovascular risks associated with non-steroidal anti-inflammatory drugs. *Lancet* 2008;371:270–3.

This chapter provides quick reference tables of management options for individual osteoarthritis (OA) joint problems (Tables 9.1–9.3). In general, all non-pharmacological options should be considered early, with some sequence or 'step-up' when using pharmacological interventions. Remember, none of these therapies is mutually exclusive and patients who are not responding should be offered as many options as possible before surgery is considered. Therapies will need to be tailored according to an individual patient's comorbidities.

Intra-articular corticosteroids

Synthetic corticosteroids are excellent anti-inflammatory agents. Intra-articular corticosteroids have been used in OA since the 1950s, although relatively few randomized controlled trials using these agents have been carried out. It is assumed that the analgesic efficacy of corticosteroids is related to their anti-inflammatory actions, although this has not been clearly demonstrated.

TABLE 9.1

Management of knee osteoarthritis

Non-pharmacological therapies

- Education/written information on OA
- Weight loss (in those who are overweight)
- Leg-strengthening exercises (see Chapter 7)
- Aerobic exercise
- Appropriate shock-absorbing footwear
- Walking aid, if an individual is in danger of falls or unresponsive to other therapies
- Review work and social activities that aggravate pain and/or may place an individual at risk of injury

CONTINUED

TABLE 9.1 (CONTINUED)

Pharmacological therapies

- Trial of regular paracetamol (acetaminophen), 1000 mg, up to three times daily
- Topical NSAIDs for short-term pain relief (usually not oral NSAIDs)
- Topical capsaicin may be added to other analgesics
- Short-term use of NSAIDs or COX-2 selective agents (consider patient risk factors; see Table 8.2, page 84)
- Intra-articular steroid injection for short-term (few weeks) pain reduction, particularly to allow exercise

  Intra-articular hyaluronan injections (though difficulty in selecting appropriate patient group based on current studies)
- Opioid analgesics (consider half-life and oral/transdermal route)

Surgical intervention

- Osteotomy in appropriate younger patients (indications for this should be discussed with the surgeon)
- Hemi-compartmental joint replacement
- Total joint replacement

Clinical hints

- Patients with fixed-flexion deformities will have difficulties with exercises
- Patients who limp or who have weak quadriceps may have associated trochanteric bursitis, which may respond to local steroid injection (to knee, trochanteric bursa or both) together with quadriceps exercises

COX, cyclooxygenase; NSAID, non-steroidal anti-inflammatory drug; OA, osteoarthritis.

As most readers will be aware, there are a number of different corticosteroid preparations but experts have not reached consensus on what dose or which particular agent should be used for a given OA joint. Methylprednisolone and triamcinolone are commonly used, the latter being a more potent steroid, although few data exist on whether

TABLE 9.2

Management of hip osteoarthritis

Non-pharmacological therapies

- Education/written information on OA
- Weight loss (in those who are overweight)
- Strengthening exercises for the hip and knee muscles
- Aerobic exercise
- Appropriate shock-absorbing footwear
- Walking aid if in danger of falls or unresponsive to other therapies
- Review work and social activities that aggravate pain and may place the individual at risk for injury

Pharmacological therapies

- Trial of regular paracetamol (acetaminophen), 1000 mg, up to three times daily
- Short-term use of NSAIDs or COX-2 selective agents (consider patient risk factors; see Table 8.2, page 84)
- Intra-articular steroid injection for short-term (few weeks) pain reduction, particularly to allow exercise
- Opioid analgesics (consider half-life and oral/transdermal route)
- Guided intra-articular steroid injection (using ultrasonography or fluoroscopy) for short-term pain reduction

Surgical intervention

- Hemi-compartmental joint replacement (including hip re-surfacing)
- Total joint replacement

Clinical hints

- In patients who present with knee pain, consider hip pathology if they have difficulty putting on shoes and socks – hip pain may refer to the knee
- Trochanteric bursitis associated with OA of the hip rarely responds well to local steroid injection

COX, cyclooxygenase; NSAID, non-steroidal anti-inflammatory drug; OA, osteoarthritis.

TABLE 9.3

Management of hand osteoarthritis

Non-pharmacological therapies

- Education/written information on OA
- Forearm strengthening exercises
- Splint for first CMC joint (base of thumb)
- Review work and social activities that aggravate pain and may place person at risk of injury

Pharmacological therapies

- Trial of regular paracetamol (acetaminophen), 1000 mg, up to three times daily.
- Topical NSAIDs for short-term pain relief (usually not with oral NSAIDs)
- Topical capsaicin may be added to other analgesics
- Short-term use of NSAIDs or COX-2 selective agents (consider patient risk factors; see Table 8.2, page 84)
- Intra-articular steroid injection for short-term pain reduction (guided injection may be more useful)
- Opioid analgesics (consider half-life and oral/transdermal route)

Surgical intervention

- Specialized surgery options for first CMC joint (base of thumb)

Clinical hints

- Small joint osteoarthritis (distal and proximal interphalangeal) is often painful for months while clinical deformity is first developing, after which the joint may be stiff but less painful
- Though not as common as distal or proximal interphalangeal involvement, OA of the metacarpophalangeal joints does occur and in the elderly is a common differential diagnosis for rheumatoid arthritis

CMC, carpometacarpal; COX, cyclooxygenase; NSAIDs, non-steroidal anti-inflammatory drugs; OA, osteoarthritis.

this provides any clinically significant differences in outcome. In general, a greater dose of drug is given into a large joint (e.g. methylprednisolone, 80 mg, for the knee versus 10 mg in the base of the thumb).

On balance, steroid injection studies show a moderate benefit in reducing symptoms for 1–3 weeks after injection. However, it should be noted that intra-articular injection may miss the joint, even when given by experts!

Indications. In OA, intra-articular steroids may be useful in patients:
- who need sufficient pain relief to perform appropriate strengthening exercises
- with a large knee effusion that interferes with function
- with a ruptured Baker's cyst (see page 56).

To facilitate exercise. Most commonly, steroid injections are administered as a pain 'circuit-breaker' to allow appropriate exercises to be performed. Patients are usually able to start exercise of the joint a few days after the injection. This can be particularly useful in patients with moderate-to-severely painful trochanteric bursitis, secondary to limping and poor quadriceps strength, where the bursitis is hampering the patient's muscle-strengthening efforts.

Large knee effusion. Although injection can be useful in patients with a large knee effusion that interferes with function, the presence of an effusion does not automatically warrant intra-articular therapy, although aspiration may be helpful.

Ruptured Baker's cyst. The patient may have been aware of a swelling or lump at the back of the knee for some time, but then will be aware of a burning sensation and swelling of the calf, perhaps in association with a flare of knee swelling. The major differential diagnosis is that of a deep venous thrombosis. As most Baker's cysts communicate with the knee joint cavity, intra-articular steroid into the knee joint often reduces fluid production and leakage from the cyst.

Number of injections. One of the most commonly asked questions in OA is: how many times can an individual joint be injected? Much of the information on this comes from animal model studies and there are no good data in humans on which to make such recommendations. A general rule of no more than three or four injections in a given year is often quoted. Certainly injection therapy should never be given as a sole therapy but combined with appropriate exercises.

Injection technique. Intra-articular injections are usually performed using an aseptic technique. They should only be undertaken under the supervision of, and after training from, a physician with expertise in the appropriate techniques. Ultrasound guidance improves injection accuracy and, potentially, patient comfort and clinical response.

Side effects. The major risk from intra-articular injection is that of septic arthritis, which is thankfully extremely uncommon when proper preparation of the site and technique are used. It is wise to warn patients that flare of joint pain may occur after injection, albeit in a small percentage of patients. This may be due to a reaction to the steroid preparation and usually settles within 24 hours. If steroid is deposited subcutaneously it can cause fat atrophy, which may cause unsightly dimples in visible areas.

One of the potential risks of intra-articular steroid injections is that of worsening OA ('steroid arthropathy'). Again, much of this concept is based on animal studies and no good clinical evidence is available to support this concept. Most patients have structural damage before injection, and subsequent monitoring of structural damage in the clinic is very difficult given current radiographic imaging (this may change with MRI monitoring). The few retrospective studies are confounded by the degree of patient symptoms and structural damage. Certainly, prolonged use of intra-articular steroid alone is not optimal management of OA and other options should be discussed with appropriate experts.

Hyaluronans

Hyaluronan (hyaluronic acid; HA) is a major non-structural component of both the synovial and cartilage extracellular matrices (see Chapter 1). It is also found in the synovial fluid. Levels in the synovial fluid of individuals with OA are reduced, which has led to a theoretical concept known as viscosupplementation – the injection of exogenous or synthesized HA into a joint to improve synovial fluid viscosity and subsequently symptoms.

Although a number of mechanisms have been proposed for the action of exogenous HA, such as beneficial effects on chondrocyte function and improving HA production by synovial fibroblasts in vitro, there are no convincing data on how HA works in humans. In particular, HA is generally cleared from the joint within 24 hours and any mechanism of action must therefore take into account the prolonged clinical benefits reported.

A variety of HA preparations of differing molecular weight and origin are available, and they are recommended with differing treatment protocols, some being used as single injections and others as 3–5 week courses of weekly injections.

Many clinical trials of HA therapy, the vast majority in OA of the knee, have been conducted. On balance, these clinical trials have demonstrated, at best, a modest benefit in reducing symptoms, starting with improvements immediately after the course of injections, peaking at around 2 months, and persisting for up to 6 months. Studies suggest that this small effect may only occur in mildly arthritic knees. Practitioners must also take into account the cost–benefits of these therapies. In the UK, the National Institute for Health and Clinical Excellence (NICE) has advised against HA therapy following a cost-effectiveness analysis.

Side effects. The most common side effect of these therapies is a post-injection flare of knee pain (sometimes with florid synovitis), which is quite uncommon. Occasionally, there can be local irritation around the injection site. As with all intra-articular therapies, there is a very small risk of infection.

Key points – joint-specific management (including injections)

- Corticosteroid joint injections provide moderate short-term pain relief in a number of joints.
- Injections should always be used in conjunction with muscle-strengthening exercises to take full advantage of the steroid-induced reduction in pain.

Key references

Bannuru RR, Natov NS, Dasi UR, et al. Therapeutic trajectory following intra-articular hyaluronic acid injection in knee osteoarthritis—meta-analysis. *Osteoarthritis Cartilage* 2011; 19:611–19.

Saunders S, Longworth S. *Injection Techniques in Orthopaedics and Sports Medicine*, 3rd edn. Oxford: Churchill Livingstone, 2006.

Speed C, Hazleman B, Dalton S. Local injection therapies. In: *Fast Facts: Soft Tissue Disorders*, 2nd edn. Oxford: Health Press Limited, 2006:41–7.

Surgery is often the final stage of treatment for many patients with arthritis. In the light of the success of surgical procedures, increasing longevity of the population and greater expectations for prolonged active lifestyles, demand for surgical interventions for OA, especially hip and knee joint replacement surgery, has risen substantially since these procedures were first undertaken approximately 40 years ago.

The aim of surgical procedures is to reduce pain and improve function; these procedures involve techniques that:
- preserve or restore joint surfaces
- replace joints with artificial implants
- fuse joints (arthrodeses).

Patient selection

The decision to consider surgical intervention should be made after conservative treatment approaches – adequate analgesia, muscle strengthening and weight loss if appropriate – have been exhausted. There is little evidence on which to base the selection of suitable candidates for surgery, and ultimately the decision for surgical referral should be made by the patient in conjunction with a relevant musculoskeletal specialist who will provide information on the benefits and risks of the particular surgical intervention.

Each case must be assessed individually, and should include an analysis of the patient's:
- severity of symptoms
- functional limitations
- general health
- expectations.

Referral decisions should not be influenced by factors such as age or sex, or other factors such as smoking and obesity, although clearly factors that are unrelated to joint pain must be taken into account, including comorbidities and concerns relating to anesthesia. Radiographic findings may add to the assessment, but do not provide a reliable basis for referral decisions, as they do not correlate perfectly with symptoms. This chapter provides a general overview of a number of relatively common procedures.

Arthroscopic debridement and lavage

Debridement of a joint refers to the procedure of smoothing off the roughened cartilage surfaces and menisci, shaving tibial spine osteophytes that may interfere with joint motion and removing inflamed synovium. Lavage – the process of 'washing out' the joint – aims to remove debris such as fragments of cartilage and calcium phosphate crystals. A substantial body of evidence, including well-designed randomized controlled trials with sham surgery controls, now indicates that arthroscopic debridement and lavage of the knee, in the absence of meniscal damage, do not provide benefits in pain or function for patients with knee OA and should not be recommended in most cases. Trials are under way to determine the role of arthroscopy in meniscal tears. Closed needle lavage or tidal irrigation may have a role, but further studies are required. Arthroscopic surgery at the hip to correct incongruency between the femoral head and acetabulum, as in femoroacetabular impingement, is increasingly performed, although little evidence exists regarding long-term outcomes or appropriate indications.

Osteotomy

Osteotomy involves excision of bone to correct joint deformity. The aim is to reduce axial malalignment and incongruency of weight-bearing surfaces that may have been caused by congenital or developmental factors, or by the effects of the OA process, thereby preventing further damage to the worn part of the joint.

This procedure is generally reserved for younger patients, and even children, in an attempt to prevent or reduce premature OA. High tibial osteotomy of the knee may be useful in younger patients with medial compartment OA and early-stage radiographic disease. The subset of individuals in whom tibial osteotomy will be beneficial in the long term is not clear, and the procedure has been performed less commonly in recent years. Evidence suggests a 25% failure rate over

10 years, with individuals often requiring knee joint replacement, but no controlled trials have been done to determine whether the procedure ultimately delays OA progression. It is worth noting that bone removal during this procedure may make subsequent joint replacement a more complex procedure. Similarly in the hip, acetabular osteotomy can be performed for dysplastic hips to reorient and 'normalize' the position of the acetabulum, although it is unknown whether this delays onset or slows progression of hip OA.

Total knee or hip replacement

Knee and hip replacements are amongst the most commonly performed surgical procedures. In 2004, it was reported that over 50 000 total hip replacements and over 30 000 knee replacements are undertaken in the UK every year; in 2006 in the US, 231 000 hip and 542 000 knee replacements were performed.

Joint replacement is arguably one of the most effective therapies for OA of the knee or hip, although the evidence for this benefit is drawn mostly from observational studies. The indications for joint replacement usually include moderate-to-severe pain that is unresponsive to conservative measures and radiographic evidence of severe OA structural damage. With modern techniques, 90% or more of hip and knee replacements function 10–20 years after surgery (risk of revision surgery of 1% per year), and approximately 90% of patients will get a good reduction in pain after joint replacement.

People referred for surgery should understand both the benefits and risks of the particular procedure. Complications are rare but may include blood clots (deep venous thrombosis of the leg), chest infection or wound infection, which may delay recovery. Most people undergoing hip or knee replacement surgery will be able to leave the hospital after an average of 3 days, although they may need to use a walking aid such as a stick for some weeks. Recovery is greatly helped by preoperative muscle conditioning and compliance with postoperative rehabilitation. Adequate analgesia in the perioperative period is essential to aid rehabilitation (although many patients may require less analgesia than preoperatively).

Expectations for postoperative activity levels should be realistic. Patients will not be able to drive or work in the first 6–8 weeks. There will be long-term restrictions in some movements and some functional limitations. Postoperative joint dislocation is uncommon, but patients need to be aware that certain positions and movements should be avoided, and that artificial hip and knee joints will not allow heavy work, lifting or repetitive impacts.

Joint-conserving surgery

Recently, a number of joint-conserving surgeries have improved. As experience grows with these procedures they may well offer opportunities to patients who are too young to be considered for joint replacement surgery.

Unicompartmental arthroplasty of the knee involves replacing of one half of the joint (medial or lateral) whilst preserving the other half. Replacement of the medial compartment of the knee is most common. Benefits of this procedure compared with total joint replacement include a smaller surgical incision, shorter length of stay in hospital and quicker rehabilitation. There is no evidence that the long-term survival of a unicompartmental knee replacement is better or worse than a total knee replacement, and the pain relief a few months after surgery is similar. This operation is growing in frequency, with longer-term follow-up data still accruing, although a 2007 Cochrane review reported 'silver' level evidence that valgus high tibial osteotomy improves knee function and reduces pain (www.cochranemsk.org).

Patella resurfacing involves the insertion of a synthetic material component in the back of the knee cap and a metal component in the front of the femur, leaving the main knee joint between the tibia and the femur intact. Patellofemoral resurfacing is a relatively new technique compared with total knee replacement, but may be indicated in people who have isolated OA of the patellofemoral joint.

Femoral head resurfacing involves replacement of the surface of the femoral head without removal of the neck of the femur. The potential advantages over total hip replacement include bone preservation and a potentially lower incidence of hip dislocation, although disadvantages include possible femoral neck fracture and high revision rates. This procedure is generally used in younger people, but anatomic factors of the hip joint are also relevant in selection of appropriate candidates for this procedure.

Tissue engineering

A number of other surgical procedures that use tissue- and cell-based repair of cartilage loss are performed in specialist centers. Techniques include chondral defect drilling, abrasion chondroplasty and microfracture – approaches that are designed to stimulate the body's own repair mechanisms to regenerate new tissue to heal the damaged or worn articular cartilage and subchondral bone.

Other methods aimed at promoting regeneration of damaged articular tissues include autologous chondrocyte implantation, involving the culture of articular cartilage 'chondral' cells that are removed from the knee and then reimplanted into the damaged area, and autologous osteochondral transplantation, involving the removal of healthy plugs of bone and articular cartilage from areas within the same joint where loading is less, and insertion into the damaged area. These techniques are highly specialized, successful tissue regeneration is inconsistent, and time to normal activity can be more than a year. To date, these procedures have generally been used for younger patients with isolated chondral defects > 3 cm² and no evidence of OA; further investigation is required to assess their place in the management of OA.

Surgery for other OA joint sites

Whilst surgery is most commonly performed for OA of the knee or hip joints, other joints may also benefit from surgical intervention.

Hand surgery. OA of the trapeziometacarpal joint is a common reason for hand surgery. This joint can be fused to eliminate motion from the problem joint, or it can be reconstructed. Reconstruction generally involves trapeziectomy (removal of the degenerate trapezium carpal bone), with insertion of soft tissue such as a rolled up tendon into the resultant gap. Sometimes a joint replacement implant is inserted, and ligament reconstruction may also be performed. Such procedures have few complications and high rates of pain relief.

Foot and ankle surgery. First metatarsophalangeal joint OA can be improved with cheilectomy (removal of osteophytes) or arthrodesis. Surgical options for OA of the ankle joint include joint fusion and joint replacement surgery. Joint replacement has the advantage of preserving some movement at the talocrural joint, but has a higher failure rate. Fusion may be equally effective in relieving pain if there is adequate movement in the neighboring joints to compensate for the fixed talocrural joint, and has fewer complications.

Shoulder surgery. Shoulder replacement has experienced the most rapid increase in frequency of any joint replacement procedure, and is the most common surgery for shoulder arthritis. It does, however, involve a prolonged rehabilitation and recovery period. Reverse shoulder arthroplasty, where the humeral compartment serves as the socket and the glenoid as the ball, may be useful for individuals without an intact rotator cuff who do not have other options. Other options include joint fusion or hemiarthroplasty, where the humeral head is replaced but the glenoid surface is preserved. Debridement and synovectomy procedures can be performed arthroscopically. Degenerative tears of the rotator cuff can also be repaired in some instances.

Key points – surgical management

- Surgery should be considered only when appropriate conservative treatment approaches have been exhausted.
- Hip and knee replacement surgery is well established and may be one of the most effective therapies for these joints.
- Other surgical techniques include joint preservation and joint fusion.
- Appropriate education, advice and rehabilitation should be provided, both preoperatively and postoperatively, for people undergoing surgery.

Key references

Brouwer RW, van Raaij TM, Bierma-Zeinstra SMA et al. Osteotomy for treating knee osteoarthritis. *Cochrane Database Syst Rev* 2007;3:CD004019.

Günther K. Surgical approaches for osteoarthritis. *Best Prac Res Clin Rheumatol* 2001;15:627–43.

Katz JN, Earp BE, Gomoll AH. Surgical management of osteoarthritis. *Arthritis Care Res* 2010;62:1220–8.

Moseley K, O'Malley NG, Petersen TJ et al. A controlled trial of arthroscopic surgery for osteoarthritis of the knee. *NEJM* 2002;347:81–8.

Segal NA, Buckwalter JA, Amendola A. Other surgical techniques for osteoarthritis. *Best Prac Res Clin Rheumatol* 2006;20:155–76.

Wajon A, Ada L, Edmunds I, Carr E. Surgery for thumb (trapeziometacarpal joint) osteoarthritis. *Cochrane Database Syst Rev* 2005;4:CD004631.

Weng HH, Fitzgerald J. Current issues in joint replacement surgery. *Curr Opin Rheumatol* 2006;18:163–9.

The development of structured care pathways

With the massive rise of symptomatic osteoarthritis (OA) due to the aging 'baby boomer' population and the increasing prevalence of obesity, healthcare systems will be placed under increasing stress to manage OA. In the UK, Department of Health directives for the planning of appropriate care pathways are already in place, based on patient self-management with aid from primary care physicians and physical therapists, with much smaller numbers of patients expected to use secondary care and surgical interventions if managed appropriately. Similarly, in the USA, a number of initiatives are being supported by the National Institutes of Health (NIH) and the Centers for Disease Control and Prevention to address the rising burden of OA at the public health level. Certainly, public and private systems will increasingly look at the structure and cost-effectiveness of OA care regimens.

Improving the OA phenotype

The ability to evaluate the whole OA joint using scoring systems that evaluate all the joint structures will allow a greater understanding of the natural history of the disease at the 'macro'-structural level, and just as importantly offers the opportunity of *targeting* specific therapies. It would be expected that therapies may be more successfully applied in individual patients if the predominant feature for that patient (e.g. synovitis or bone) were targeted. The use of MRI to determine patient outcome in clinical trials will aid this process. An understanding of an individual's whole body burden of OA in multiple joints may also be useful in identifying potential treatments.

At present a number of large OA knee cohorts with MRI evaluations are in progress; in particular, the NIH Osteoarthritis Initiative will provide substantial data to inform our understanding of the natural history of this common process.

Perhaps more excitingly, MRI offers the opportunity to use functional techniques to expand our understanding of OA. T2-

mapping can examine changes in water and collagen content and collagen fibril orientation in articular cartilage. Delayed gadolinium-enhanced MRI of cartilage (dGEMRIC) is a procedure that takes advantage of the diffusion of negatively charged gadolinium contrast agent (commonly used for highlighting areas of inflammation or synovitis) into areas of articular cartilage with low levels of the negatively charged glycosaminoglycans. This procedure allows us to identify loss of glycosaminoglycans in very early OA. As the reliability of these procedures and their use as outcome measures improve, they may be crucial in assessing the efficacy of structure-modifying drugs, many of which may work only at the earliest stages of cartilage loss, before massive bone damage and abnormal biomechanical forces render drug therapy unrealistic.

The increasing use of ultrasonography may be a valuable addition to the assessment of OA joints and, more particularly, in correct placement of intra-articular therapies. This should improve response to therapies such as intra-articular corticosteroid injections, and may also be useful for future intra-articular delivery of gene therapy.

Early intervention

It makes sense to consider that both analgesia and potential structure modification may be more effective in early OA. However, there is no consensus on what constitutes 'early' clinical OA, and the use of sensitive imaging has further confounded this area. Trials will need to consider careful definitions of OA so that concepts of early intervention can be explored.

Symptomatic therapies

Optimizing current therapies. There are clearly many gaps in the current literature on OA therapies. Establishing the most time-efficient home exercise program and improving adherence to exercise therapies are key issues. Importantly, very little research has been undertaken on the effects of combining treatments; for example, do combinations of NSAIDs and opioids work better than the individual agents? In a therapeutic area where there have been few major breakthroughs, optimizing existing options seems an urgent priority.

New symptomatic therapies. Many new analgesic agents are in development, though often for indications of 'musculoskeletal pain', and it may take further time to see if such drugs work in OA. As synovitis and inflammation are important in OA pain, a range of anti-cytokine and anti-inflammatory molecules are being investigated in early phase studies for analgesic efficacy. The toxicity associated with many current therapies for OA pain has led to increased focus on pain pathways and consideration of both central and peripheral components as potential targets for intervention. One novel development is the field of nerve growth factor, a mediator that has demonstrated elevated levels in both animal and human pain models and is associated with increased hyperalgesia. Monoclonal antibodies to nerve growth factor and its receptor were successfully employed in preclinical models and have demonstrated good results in terms of pain relief in phase III trials; perhaps not surprisingly given the mechanism of action, peripheral neuropathies were (uncommon) side effects. However, further trials were halted in the USA because of safety concerns after increased rates of joint replacement were observed. Investigations are under way to determine if these are drug- or class-specific effects or may relate to increased weight-bearing through critically damaged OA joints.

Preliminary data presented at the Osteoarthritis Research Society International (OARSI) annual meeting in 2011 on a proprietary formulation of oral salmon calcitonin suggested improvements in WOMAC pain (see page 66), physical function, and stiffness over the 2-year trial period. Although the primary endpoint (radiographic joint space width) was not reached, there were small improvements in MRI cartilage volume.

Structure-modifying therapies

Structure modification may involve surgical intervention (such as in the ankle and knee where there are some reports of joint distraction operations resulting in structural radiographic improvements), but the main focus to date in this field has been on the development of pharmacological therapies. The aim of an ideal OA therapy is to normalize or substantially improve the structural OA pathology and to prevent further deterioration; it has always been assumed that if such therapies were successful, they would be associated with reduced symptoms and/or reduced symptom progression. This is a key issue as current regulatory approval requires modification of both OA structure (as assessed by measuring joint-space width on radiographs) and symptoms; there are no agents currently approved as disease-modifying OA drugs (DMOADs). It is possible to conceptualize that a structure-modifying therapy may not affect symptoms (e.g. by an effect on aneural cartilage alone) and it will be interesting to see how this view may evolve, especially in light of improved structural quantification with modern imaging.

Various agents have reported evidence of structure modification. In a large trial, the tetracycline doxycycline had some effect on reducing radiographic joint-space loss in the target (study) knee, but it did not change joint space in the contralateral knee and it had no effects on symptoms. Glucosamine sulfate has reported beneficial effects on joint-space narrowing but methodological issues about how radiographs were performed in these studies mean further trials will be required. A range of novel agents are in development with the potential for modifying OA structural pathology, including anti-cytokine therapies and inhibitors of matrix metalloproteinases and aggrecanases.

Joint distraction. Recent work from the Netherlands suggests that distraction of the tibiofemoral joint using an external fixation frame for 2 months results in increased joint-space width and cartilage thickness, and reduced denuded bone area. Positive trends in biomarkers, WOMAC and visual analog pain scores were also noted in this small pilot study, with prolonged benefits to at least 2 years of follow up. Understanding of the potential mechanisms of action of this therapy may provide highly important insights into in vivo repair mechanisms, opening up a new range of therapies.

Stem-cell therapy. The use of autologous chondrocyte transplantation was mentioned in Chapter 10 (page 100). Other cells also have the capability to differentiate into chondrocytes, the key cells of interest being adult mesenchymal stem cells. These pluripotent cells not only differentiate into chondrocytes but also into bone, muscle and fat cells. These cells may be found in the bone marrow but also in the synovial fluid of patients with OA. The use of such cells in regenerative medicine is a keenly watched area of development. Issues here include:

- obtaining appropriate precursor cells
- ensuring differentiation into chondrocytes
- coping with inflammation at the site of existing OA, which may interfere with cell adherence and the differentiation process
- the types of matrix that the cells will be embedded in within a cartilage defect.

This is certainly an exciting area of OA research.

Gene therapy. There are a large number of candidate genes that may be modified in the OA process. Recent studies demonstrate improved gene transfer at the specific joint level. It is hoped that some of the exciting work showing suppression of inflammation in animal models, with subsequent reduction in progression of cartilage lesions (e.g. using the interleukin-1 receptor antagonist gene), may be applied in OA in humans.

Key references

Hunter DJ. Pharmacologic therapy for osteoarthritis—the era of disease modification. *Nat Rev Rheumatol* 2011;7:13–22.

Intema F, Van Roermund PM, Marijnissen ACA et al. Tissue structure modification in knee osteoarthritis by use of joint distraction: an open 1-year pilot study. *Ann Rheum Dis* 2011; 70:1441–6.

Karsdal MA, Alexandersen P, John MR et al. Oral calcitonin demonstrated symptom-modifying efficacy and increased cartilage volume: results from a 2-year phase 3 trial in patients with osteoarthritis of the knee. *Osteoarthritis Cartilage* 2011;19(suppl 1):S35 abstr.

Lane NE, Schnitzer TJ, Birbara CA et al. Tanezumab for the treatment of pain from osteoarthritis of the knee. *N Engl J Med* 2010;363: 1521–31.

Useful resources

UK
Arthritis Care
Tel: +44 (0)20 7380 6500
info@arthritiscare.org.uk
www.arthritiscare.org.uk

Arthritis and Musculoskeletal Alliance
Tel: +44 (0)20 7842 0910/11
www.arma.uk.net

Arthritis Research UK
Tel: +44 (0)300 790 0400
enquiries@arthritisresearchuk.org
www.arthritisresearchuk.org

British Orthopaedic Association
Tel: +44 (0)20 7405 6507
www.boa.ac.uk

British Society for Rheumatology
Tel: +44 (0)20 7842 0900
bsr@rheumatology.org.uk
www.rheumatology.org.uk

Primary Care Rheumatology Society
Tel: +44 (0)1609 774794
helen@pcrsociety.org
www.pcrsociety.org

USA
American College of Rheumatology
Tel: +1 404 633 3777
acr@rheumatology.org
www.rheumatology.org

American Orthopaedic Association
Tel: +1 847 318 7330
info@aoassn.org
www.aoassn.org

Arthritis Foundation
Toll-free: 1 800 283 7800
www.arthritis.org

International
Arthritis Australia
Toll-free: 1 800 011 041
Tel: +61 (0)2 9518 4441
info@arthritisaustralia.com.au
www.arthritisaustralia.com.au

Australian Rheumatology Association
Tel: +61 (0)2 9256 5458
robynm@racp.edu.au
www.rheumatology.org.au

Canadian Rheumatology
Association
Tel: +1 905 952 0698
cra@rogers.com
www.rheum.ca

European League Against
Rheumatism
Tel: +41 44 716 30 30
eular@eular.org
www.eular.org

Osteoarthritis Research Society
International
Tel: +1 856 439 1385
oarsi@oarsi.org
www.oarsi.org

Other useful titles

Borenstein DG, Calin A. *Fast Facts:
Low Back Pain*, 2nd edn. Oxford:
Health Press Limited, 2012.

Cousins MJ, Gallagher RM. *Fast Facts:
Chronic and Cancer Pain*, 2nd edn.
Oxford: Health Press Limited, 2011.

Compston JE, Rosen CJ. *Fast Facts:
Osteoporosis*, 6th edn. Oxford: Health
Press Limited, 2009.

Isaacs JD, Moreland LW. *Fast Facts:
Rheumatoid Arthritis*, 2nd edn.
Oxford: Health Press Limited, 2011.

Speed C, Hazleman B, Dalton S. *Fast
Facts: Soft Tissue Disorders*, 2nd edn.
Oxford: Health Press Limited, 2006.

Patient Pictures – Clinical drawings for
your patients
patientpictures.com/rheum

Index